T0175531

HANDBOOK OF
Good Psychiatric Management for Borderline Personality Disorder

HANDBOOK OF
Good Psychiatric Management for Borderline Personality Disorder

By

John G. Gunderson, M.D.
Professor of Psychiatry, Harvard Medical School;
Director, BPD Center for Treatment, Research and Training,
McLean Hospital, Belmont, Massachusetts

With

Paul S. Links, M.D., M.Sc., F.R.C.P.C.
Professor and Chair, Department of Psychiatry,
Schulich School of Medicine and Dentistry,
The University of Western Ontario;
Chief of Psychiatry, London Health Sciences Centre
and St. Joseph's Health Care, London, Ontario

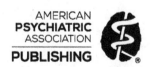

AMERICAN
PSYCHIATRIC
ASSOCIATION
PUBLISHING

Note: The authors have worked to ensure that all information in this book is accurate at the time of publication and consistent with general psychiatric and medical standards, and that information concerning drug dosages, schedules, and routes of administration is accurate at the time of publication and consistent with standards set by the U.S. Food and Drug Administration and the general medical community. As medical research and practice continue to advance, however, therapeutic standards may change. Moreover, specific situations may require a specific therapeutic response not included in this book. For these reasons and because human and mechanical errors sometimes occur, we recommend that readers follow the advice of physicians directly involved in their care or the care of a member of their family.

Books published by American Psychiatric Association Publishing (APAP) represent the findings, conclusions, and views of the individual authors and do not necessarily represent the policies and opinions of APAP or the American Psychiatric Association.

If you wish to buy 50 or more copies of the same title, please go to www.appi.org/specialdiscounts for more information..

Copyright © 2014 American Psychiatric Association
ALL RIGHTS RESERVED

Manufactured in the United States of America on acid-free paper
26   25   24   23   22   11   10   9   8   7
First Edition

Typeset in Adobe's Warnock Pro and Trade Gothic LT Std.

American Psychiatric Association Publishing
800 Maine Avenue SW, Suite 900
Washington, DC 20024-2812
www.appi.org

Library of Congress Cataloging-in-Publication Data
Gunderson, John G., 1942– author.
 Handbook of good psychiatric management for borderline personality disorder / by John G. Gunderson ; with Paul S. Links. — First edition.
     p. ; cm.
 Includes bibliographical references and index.
 ISBN 978-1-58562-460-7 (pbk. : alk. paper)
 I. Links, Paul S., author. II. American Psychiatric Publishing, issuing body. III. Title.
 [DNLM: 1. Borderline Personality Disorder—therapy—Handbooks. 2. Evidence-Based Practice—methods—Handbooks. WM 34]
 RC569.5.B67
 616.85'852—dc23

                                                              2013044898

British Library Cataloguing in Publication Data
A CIP record is available from the British Library.

Contents

Preface vii

Acknowledgments. xi

SECTION I
Background

1 Introduction to
Good Psychiatric Management (GPM) 3

SECTION II
GPM Manual
Treatment Guidelines

2 Overall Principles. 13

3 Making the Diagnosis 21

4 Getting Started 27

5 Managing Suicidality
and Nonsuicidal Self-Harm 37

6 Pharmacotherapy and Comorbidity. 47

7 Split Treatments 57

SECTION III
GPM Workbook
Case Illustrations

8 **Case Illustrations** **71**

SECTION IV
GPM Video Guide
Demonstrations of the Approach

9 **Video Demonstrations** **143**

    Videos online at www.appi.org/Gunderson

Appendix A **145**

    Relation of Good Psychiatric Management to
    Other Evidence-Based Treatments for
    Borderline Personality Disorder

Appendix B **149**

    Common Features of Evidence-Based Treatments
    for Borderline Personality Disorder

Appendix C **151**

    Safety Planning: An Example

Appendix D **153**

    Guidelines for Families

References **157**

Index **161**

Preface

Patients with borderline personality disorder (BPD) constitute about 20% of inpatient and outpatient clinic patients. Yet in an era when costs of health care are soaring, the care provided to them is extremely inconsistent in quality and, worse, can easily be harmful. Borderline patients have a right to expect better or, at the very least, to expect that the mental health professionals responsible for their care have received basic training.

Regrettably, the training of most professionals is provided solely by their individual supervisors, who themselves have had no BPD-specific training. Training programs typically include little didactic information about BPD's psychopathology, let alone about evidence-based practices. Most professionals will readily admit that their training was insufficient for them to feel comfortable about, and capable of, treating BPD. To some extent, this lack of training and this lack of confidence are symptomatic of a collective countertransference within the mental health and medical fields; most psychiatrists and other physicians don't like and actively avoid borderline patients ("Borderline Personality: The Disorder That Doctors Fear Most," *Time* magazine cover story, January 19, 2009 [Cloud 2009]; Shanks et al. 2011). Of course, it is not just countertransference. In part, the negative attitudes about treating these patients are a result of persisting myths about what such treatments are thought to require (see table, overleaf). Unfortunately, also looming behind the lack of training, enthusiasm, and self-confidence by treaters is the reality that borderline patients can be difficult. Borderline patients actively challenge the hard-earned authority and the skill set professionals have been proud to attain.

Although these perspectives can help explain our profession's persisting failure to provide basic training, they do not justify it. It is time for mental health professionals to embrace the challenge posed by these patients. Borderline personality disorder will not allow us to ignore them. We have the knowledge to master the challenge and to be rewarded for having done so.

The purpose of this handbook is to provide the means through which psychiatrists and other mental health professionals can become "good

Myths about treatment of borderline personality disorder (BPD)

Myth	Clarification
BPD patients resist treatment.	Most actively seek relief from subjective pain; treatment for their personality disorder requires psychoeducation by clinicians.
BPD patients angrily attack their treaters.	Excessive anger and fearful wariness toward others, especially caregivers, are symptoms (i.e., instinctive transferences) of their disorder.
BPD patients rarely get better.	About 10% remit within 6 months, 25% by a year, and 50% by 2 years. Once patients have remitted, relapses are unusual.
BPD patients get better only if given extended, intensive treatment by experts.	Such treatment is required by only a subsample. Most do well within intermittent treatment by well-meaning nonexperts. Intense treatments can easily become regressive.
Recurrent risk of suicide invariably burdens treaters with serious liability risks.	Excessive burden or fears of litigation are symptoms of inexperience and of treatments that are poorly structured.
Recurrent crises require treaters to be available 24/7.	Such a requirement is rare and usually means that a different level or type of care is needed.

enough" to treat most cases of BPD competently and to take satisfaction from having done this well.

Splits are part of us all. Relationships with patients with BPD provide fertile soil for our internal splits to blossom. Only in retrospect have I recognized how my first reactions to these patients were so much governed by my negative fears of being controlled or seduced that those reactions had overwhelmed my positive hopes to protect and nurture. So I defensively went about the business of learning how to establish boundaries, recognize my borderline patients' covert anger, and prevent regressions. Of course, learning these lessons involved many mistakes, hurt feelings, and failed or, more commonly, abruptly shortened treatments. It also led to regrets, apologies, and humility. I grew self-conscious about my Calvinistic presence.

As my defensive fears of being intruded upon receded, my wishes to protect and be appreciated emerged. I worked at listening, validating, and being empathic, and in this process, I began to experience uninvited feelings of compassion and tenderness. I learned that it was an achievement for my BPD patients to be able to trust and depend on me. Clinicians who can contain defensive reactions toward their borderline patients and who can learn compassion toward them are well prepared to be helpful. The basic principles of Good Psychiatric Management (GPM) developed primarily from clinical experience and the personal growth that was required.

Treaters who practice GPM are encouraged to be active agents in helping borderline patients understand their inner experience, in reshaping their behavioral adaptations, and in establishing a good life. This treatment comfortably utilizes cognitive, behavioral, and psychodynamic interventions. As will be evident in this text, GPM borrows heavily from concepts introduced earlier by Winnicott (1953) such as "holding environment" and "good enough" parenting. These concepts decry too much specificity or perfectionism; they fit comfortably with GPM's emphasis on the borderline patient's interpersonal hypersensitivity (see Chapter 2 ["Overall Principles"]) and with a dyadic model of the therapy relationships.

Many years of trial-and-error experience forged this handbook's case management practices, which are practical and pragmatic. In retrospect, most of what I learned seems quite obvious. I hope that readers will find this to be true for them. I do not see myself as particularly gifted, and I do not believe that only experts can be effective treaters. I do believe that I have become "good enough" for most borderline patients and that if I can do this work, then so can most others.

John Gunderson

Acknowledgments

As this book's primary author, I am responsible for whatever is speculative or proves misleading. In contrast, Paul Links, M.D., M.Sc., F.R.C.P.C., my long-standing colleague, is responsible for containing my excesses, for sharpening this book's messages, and for contributing his wise and practical clinical insights. Perhaps even more essentially, he can be held responsible for triggering the writing of this book. Had he not taken the initiative, invested his skills, and had the audacity to test, then confirm, the efficacy of a treatment called Good Psychiatric Management (GPM) (McMain et al. 2009) heavily modeled on what I had written, I would have been content to have my clinical perspectives remain the province of scholar and able supervisor. When GPM proved efficacious, it suggested that my clinical perspectives might offer a standard of care that should be more broadly taught. Hence this book.

Many others have contributed to the development of this book's case illustrations (Section III: GPM Workbook) and videos (Section IV: GPM Video Guide). Specifically, the following colleagues helped prepare the following case illustrations: Case 1—Brian Palmer, M.D.; Case 3—Brad Reich, M.D.; and Case 4—Lois Choi-Kain, M.D. Claire Brickell, M.D., suggested changes in all of the case illustrations and helped identify how they showed GPM's basic principles. The seemingly endless process of revising this book's contents was patiently overseen by my secretary, Linda DeVito Ghilardi.

The following colleagues helped prepare the videos: Video 2, "Diagnostic Disclosure"—Brian Palmer, M.D.; Video 5, "Managing Safety"—Paul Links, M.D., M.Sc., F.R.C.P.C., and Amy Gagliardi, M.D.; Video 6, "Managing Anger"—Claire Brickell, M.D.; and Video 8, "Managing Safety and Medications"—Paul Links, M.D., M.Sc., F.R.C.P.C. The video editing reflects the talents of Michael Williams from McLean's Materials Management Department. The patients were all "pseudopatients," artfully portrayed by members of McLean Hospital except for one from the Mayo Clinic (Video 2) and one from the Department of Psychiatry, University of Western Ontario, London, Ontario (Video 8).

Since this handbook's initial draft, parts of it have been presented to many audiences. Each presentation has prompted revisions that have improved the book. Of particular note has been the opportunity of presenting each part of this book to colleagues at McLean Hospital. The breadth of their perspectives (from psychoanalytic to behavioral) and the depth of their clinical experience have forced me to reconsider, clarify, and sometimes omit sections that could not stand up to the test of their critiques. I am most seriously indebted to this rare collegial community for both stimulating and sharing what I have learned about treating borderline personality disorder.

J.G.

Disclosure: *The authors affirm that they have no financial interests or affiliations that present or could appear to present a conflict of interest with regard to the content and publication of this book.*

SECTION I

Background

CHAPTER 1

Introduction to
Good Psychiatric Management (GPM)

This handbook is prescriptive: what to do, how to do it, and what not to do. It provides guides to turn to when one is unsure how to proceed with treatment. It recurrently encourages treaters to educate their patients about the disorder, most especially about the role of an inherited disposition and what is the expectable course. The interventions being recommended are meant to be commonsensical and simple to implement.

Section II, "GPM Manual: Treatment Guidelines," provides a condensed and clear description of the most essential and specific interventions in Good Psychiatric Management (GPM). It can be used as a guide for research from which measures of adherence and competence are available (Kolla et al. 2009). But, unlike a true manual, this handbook was not primarily written to ensure adherence so that efficacy can be tested. It does not proscribe "off-model" interventions; it recognizes that good clinical care is inherently flexible, pragmatic, and adapted to each patient. Its primary purpose is to describe clinical practices that clinicians can learn from and use in everyday practice. To facilitate this, Section III, "GPM Workbook: Case Illustrations," offers case vignettes interrupted by "decision points." At each of these decision points, different interventions are proposed and discussed. To further facilitate learning, Section IV, "GPM Video Guide: Demonstrations of the Approach," describes a set of nine videotaped interactions that can be viewed online. Here readers can see in vivo illustrations of the GPM model in practice.

Impelling this handbook's preparation was the vision that with adequate training, most psychiatrists and other mental health professionals can become "good enough" to treat most cases of BPD competently and to take satisfaction in a job well done. You don't need to be a specialist, to be selflessly devoted, or to have a larger-than-life personality to be "good enough"; you do need to be warm, reliable, interested, and unintimidated. and you need basic knowledge about case management. That is where this handbook comes in; if you know enough to avoid being harmful, you can be, surprisingly, very helpful. Such knowledge has typically been acquired by several years of work on inpatient services—a setting that provides unique opportunities to witness how borderline patients' behavior and moods are exquisitely sensitive to their social context and, most notably, how reactive they are to interpersonal events. This book is intended to condense and expedite such learning.

This handbook is designed to be a basic text for all hospital, outpatient clinic, or office-based psychiatrists or mental health professionals who need to assume primary responsibility for the treatment of BPD. It is particularly apt for psychiatric residents. GPM is a pragmatic, therapeutically effective approach emphasizing case management. It should not be considered as another form of individual psychotherapy—however, like good psychotherapies, it is guided by an understanding of the psychology of borderline psychopathology. More than most psychotherapies, it embraces neurobiological (genetic and pharmacotherapeutic) and social situational (stressors, family environment, and vocational) perspectives. It also embraces the perspective of positive psychology: GPM encourages patients to pursue satisfactory and meaningful lives. Because a large proportion of borderline patients are first seen by physicians within primary care and emergency department settings, the dos and don'ts of prescribing medications offer lessons that can prevent much burden and misuse. Some sections will be especially relevant to clinicians who do individual psychotherapy. Others provide the basic what-you-need-to-know for those who specialize in substance abuse, medication-resistant depression, and consultation-liaison psychiatry.

GPM's Place in Treatment Planning

GPM is "good enough" for most borderline patients. It can be used to expedite attaining competence and satisfaction from treating BPD. It is not meant to guide long-term outpatient psychotherapy. Short-term, intermittent, and nonintensive therapies are normative and are usually "good enough" (Bender et al. 2006). Within this approach, life's lessons can become a great ally in bringing about change if they become integrated. Treaters facilitate learning these lessons.

GPM is not meant to replace or compete with evidence-based therapies such as Dialectical Behavior Therapy (DBT; Linehan 1993), Mentalization-

Based Treatment (MBT; Bateman and Fonagy 2012), Transference-Focused Psychotherapy (TFP; Yeomans et al. 2002), and Schema-Focused Therapy (SFT; Young 1990). These evidence-based treatments are intended for professionals who self-select because they want to develop expertise (i.e., they want to specialize in treating, and especially in doing extended individual psychotherapy for, BPD). For these evidence-based treatments, patients are expected to attend regular sessions, usually for 2 or more hours per week for a year or more. These treatments can be adapted for specialized BPD clinical services at tertiary facilities such as McLean Hospital (www.mclean.harvard.edu). Because of the extensive training required to attain competence in these evidence-based BPD-specific therapies and because of the commitment in time and costs they require, these therapies are rarely available. Given the estimated 2% community prevalence of BPD (i.e., in the United States, that means about 6 million people), the BPD-specific psychotherapies cannot be expected to meet the needs for their treatment. (See Appendix A, "Relation of Good Psychiatric Management to Other Evidence-Based Treatments for Borderline Personality Disorder," for further consideration of how GPM compares with these other evidence-based treatments.)

GPM offers a more basic approach to treatment of BPD than do prior evidence-based therapies, it is more suitable for initial "entry-level" training, and it contains what every primary BPD treater should know. It clearly and directly includes the perspectives of a genetic disposition and an expectation of improvement. This approach can be integrated into the standardized training curriculum by departments of psychiatry or psychology. Those patients who fail to respond to GPM or who—having been stabilized by GPM—still want better self-regulation or self-awareness are good candidates for the more intensive and extended evidence-based treatments cited above. (Such an instance is described in Chapter 8 ["Case Illustrations"]: Case 5, Lawrence.) Although these prior BPD-specific psychotherapies dramatically differ in theory and interventions, they are all comparably effective (Gabbard 2007). This conclusion has drawn attention to the therapeutic value of their common features (see Appendix B, "Common Features of Evidence-Based Treatments for Borderline Personality Disorder"). Because GPM emphasizes these common features, it will often prove capable of producing the same basic changes effected by its more rigorously defined and austerely constraining predecessors.

GPM's Precedents and Foundations

There have been many precedents from which GPM has drawn. Most notably, it is drawn from the first author's lifetime of experience in treating

BPD—experience previously documented in a series of books (Gunderson 1984, 2001; Gunderson and Links 2008). Even the first of these books (Gunderson 1984) described the basic practicalities of managing patients with BPD across modalities and levels of care as well as introducing the interpersonal focus that remains constant in GPM. Others have pioneered advocacy for the long-underappreciated value of supportive (Rockland 1987, 1992) and pragmatic (Dawson and MacMillan 1993) interventions in the treatment of BPD. GPM proudly integrates those perspectives.

Longitudinal research showing frequent, dramatic, and enduring improvements in borderline patients who did *not* receive extended or intensive therapies, much less evidence-based BPD-specific treatments, offers convincing evidence that short-term or intermittent treatment interventions can have enduring benefits (Gunderson et al. 2011; Zanarini et al. 2010). Particularly relevant was the finding that a significant number remitted within 6 months with the help of brief interventions (Gunderson et al. 2003). Two decades ago after his seminal longitudinal research, McGlashan (1993) reached a similar conclusion that borderline patients can benefit from short-term, intermittent, as-needed interventions. Notably, this research also documented the relatively poor outcomes of BPD patients in the areas of work and stable partnerships, thereby drawing attention to an area of outcome largely unaddressed by BPD's established treatments.

The randomized controlled trials that have documented the value of BPD-specific psychotherapies also lend strength to GPM's claims for effectiveness. These studies originally used weak, unregulated "treatment as usual" comparators, but in three recent trials, comparison treatments that have performed very well are markedly GPM-like. Specifically, GPM can claim marked similarities to the Expressive-Supportive (Clarkin et al. 2007), Structured Clinical Management (Bateman and Fonagy 2009), and Good Clinical Care (Chanen et al. 2008) treatments, which each did as well as TFP, MBT, and Cognitive Analytic Therapy (CAT), respectively, in almost every area of outcome. These results yielded further support for our thesis; GPM-like control treatments can do as well as their more celebrated index treatment comparators.

As shown in Table 1–1, GPM is a treatment model that is quite distinct from other evidence-based treatments by virtue of its emphasis on the interpersonal sources of emotional and behavioral symptoms and its use of psychoeducation (including discussions of genetic contributions and expectable change) and because it actively and flexibly encourages multimodal interventions. It also has the advantages of having incorporated concepts, approaches, and specific forms of intervention emphasized within other treatment models (see Table 1–2). In this sense, it is a second-generation treatment model that has selectively pruned and adapted contributions by

TABLE 1–1.   **Distinctive characteristics of GPM**

Element	Distinctive features
Case management	Focus is on the patient's life outside therapy, not primarily on the patient's psychology as in psychotherapies.
Psychoeducation	Patients and families are informed of borderline personality disorder's genetic disposition, expectable changes, and the relative merits of different approaches.
Goals	Symptom reduction and self-control are secondary goals required to attain the primary goals of success in work and partnerships.
Multimodality	Psychopharmacological practices are integrated as adjunctive alongside endorsements for group therapies and family coaching.
Duration and intensity	No specific length and intensity are prescribed; patients and therapist collaborate in judging whether a therapy is effective.
Interpersonal hypersensitivity	An explicit and consistent effort is made to connect the patient's emotions and behaviors to interpersonal stressors.

others, hopefully into a more pragmatic, generalizable, and user-friendly model.

In 2001, the "Practice Guideline for the Treatment of Patients With Borderline Personality Disorder" developed by the American Psychiatric Association (American Psychiatric Association Practice Guidelines 2001) offered a summary that overlaps with this handbook's content and intent. GPM offers considerably more emphasis on case management and less emphasis on individual psychotherapy than did the American Psychiatric Association guidelines. This handbook updates information included in a previous book by Gunderson and Links (2008) but does not purport to be as comprehensive. It adds empirically validated specificity about interventions within a specific (i.e., interpersonal hypersensitivity) model. Most significantly, this book includes two types of case-based material to facilitate training. The first is a series of case illustrations with discussions about the variety of responses clinicians might deploy in managing BPD. The second is a set of online videotaped interventions. In general, this book serves a function and proposes a treatment approach that overlaps with many precedents but remains unique and original.

TABLE 1–2.   **GPM's integration of prior evidence-based psychotherapies**

Modality	Element
Transference-Focused Psychotherapy	
Concepts	Splitting and projection as defenses against anger
Therapeutic stance	Monitoring boundaries and countertransference
Interventions	Interpretation of anger; challenge avoidance and acting out
Dialectical Behavior Therapy	
Concepts	Social and psychological skill deficits
Therapeutic stance	Coaching
Interventions	Self-monitoring; homework; intersession availability
Mentalization-Based Treatment	
Concepts	Theory of mind; attachment
Therapeutic stance	Not-knowing
Interventions	Examining attributions about self and others

GPM's Empirical Validation

In 2009, McMain et al. published a report of a large multisite randomized controlled trial showing that the clinical efficacy of General Psychiatric Management equaled that of DBT.

The "General" Psychiatric Management used in that trial can be considered the research "brand name" for the "Good" Psychiatric Management described in this book. The efficacy of General Psychiatric Management found in that study justifies the name change used here. GPM combined a psychodynamically informed case management based on the authors' previous book, *Borderline Personality Disorder: A Clinical Guide* (Gunderson and Links 2008), with the symptom-targeted medication algorithm suggested in the American Psychiatric Association Practice Guidelines (2001). This was a large single-blind multisite trial in which 180 patients diagnosed with borderline personality disorder who had at least two suicidal or nonsuicidal self-injurious episodes in the past 5 years were randomly assigned to receive 1 year of either DBT or GPM. Therapists in the GPM cell were psychiatrists (there was one psychologist) with aptitude, interest, and an average of 5 years' experience working with borderline patients. They met with the project's coinvestigator (Paul S. Links, M.D., M.Sc., F.R.C.P.C.) weekly for 6 months before the project to discuss GPM's principles and then for weekly peer supervision for the duration of the trial. Therapists in the DBT cell were primarily psychologists with prior training in DBT who met weekly with the project's Principal Investigator, Shelley McMain, as their consultation group leader throughout the project. Adherence to both treatments was established and sustained.

Both groups showed similar levels of improvement on a variety of clinical outcome measures, including significant reductions in the frequency and severity of suicidal and nonsuicidal self-injurious episodes; significant reductions in health care use, including emergency department visits and psychiatric hospital days; and significant improvements in BPD symptoms, symptom distress, depression, anger, and interpersonal functioning. No significant difference across any of these outcomes was found between the two treatments. A 2-year follow-up showed that patients sustained the gains made on suicidal and other self-injurious behaviors, health care use, and psychopathology (McMain et al. 2012). At 3 years, 62% of the patients in both groups had remitted to fewer than two criteria for a year or more, a rate that was 20% higher than for borderline patients who did not receive these BPD-specific therapies (Gunderson et al. 2011). These results indicated that a moderately well-specified treatment delivered by experienced psychiatrists who were guided by the principles described in this handbook could be highly effective—as effective as was treatment with high-quality DBT.

Although the *General* Psychiatric Management manual used during that trial rested heavily on *Borderline Personality Disorder: A Clinical Guide* (Gunderson and Links 2008), some distinctions are found between the General Psychiatric Management conducted in that trial and the *Good* Psychiatric Management guidelines offered here. One difference is that the "General" research brand was designed to be 1 year long to be comparable to DBT and thereby required informed consent involving the expectation of a 1-year commitment. The duration of "Good" Psychiatric Management as described here is pragmatic—as long as useful. Moreover, the General Psychiatric Management therapists were already experienced and liked working with borderline patients. This handbook reflects some of what those experienced psychiatrists had already learned to do, but it is intended to help less experienced treaters gain that level of competence more quickly. The third and potentially more substantive difference is that the General Psychiatric Management brand gave more hierarchical emphasis to self-harm and processing emotion than does this handbook. Those emphases may have diminished the distinctions from DBT. The model used for the

"General" research brand was that suicidal and other self-harming behaviors were mediated by problems with emotional control or processing. GPM treaters thus attempted to enhance awareness, identification, and acceptance of feeling states. The GPM described in this handbook has these same goals but ties the control of both self-harm and emotions to interpersonal stressors and to the mediating role of having a sustained and trustworthy ally via the GPM treater. A fourth difference is that "Good" PM gives a more explicit emphasis to the personal accountability, and to the goals of achieving both vocational satisfaction and stable partnerships, than did the General Psychiatric Management manual. How the study's psychiatrists actually managed this is unknown. It was clear that the "General" research brand, like all other evidence-based therapies for BPD, was not particularly effective in social or vocational rehabilitation. It is hoped that the added emphasis given here might improve that area of outcome. Finally, whereas the General Psychiatric Management brand used the American Psychiatric Association Practice Guidelines (2001) algorithm as a framework for medications (although clinicians participating in the research trial frequently departed from that algorithm on the basis of post-2001 research), in this handbook we formally propose an updated algorithm that integrates subsequent research. It is unclear whether and how any or all of these differences are significant, but, for clarity, they are highlighted here.

The results from the McMain et al. (2009) study endorse the idea that well-informed clinicians without the extensive BPD-specific training required for DBT, MBT, TFP, CAT, or SFT can provide excellent care. The research-based endorsement of GPM underscores the hope that many psychiatrists and other mental health professionals who now greet the prospect of treating BPD with unrealistic fears about their ability to be helpful can become self-confident and effective treaters.

SECTION II

GPM Manual
Treatment Guidelines

CHAPTER 2
Overall Principles

Good Psychiatric Management Theory: Interpersonal Hypersensitivity

See Video 1, Psychoeducation
Video 4, Managing Intersession Availability

In Good Psychiatric Management (GPM), the construct of interpersonal hypersensitivity explains borderline psychopathology and informs its interventions (Gunderson 2007; Gunderson and Lyons-Ruth 2008). Borderline personality disorder (BPD) phenomenology shifts dramatically in response to the person's interpersonal context (see Figure 2–1). Within treatment settings, borderline patients frequently vacillate between feeling connected or "held" when they are appealing and compliant, and feeling threatened by perceived hostility or rejection when many of their diagnostically specific feelings and behaviors (e.g., anger, self-harm) become evident. Clinicians who respond supportively will calm their patients, whereas those who respond with anger or withdrawal will activate more distressed and potentially dangerous responses.

Within ongoing relationships, clinicians (or others) can create a "holding environment" (i.e., the patient develops the containing belief that he or she is cared for) by being concerned, consistent, responsive, nonpunitive, curious, nonreactive, and uncertain. Through such experiences of feeling cared for, the borderline patient's negative sense of self can shift toward a sense of self as worthy, good, and lovable (I'm okay, i.e., "not bad," "good enough") and feeling understood (I'm understandable, coherent, not alien). This sense of self as "good enough" can become internalized from a sustained and consistent partnership.

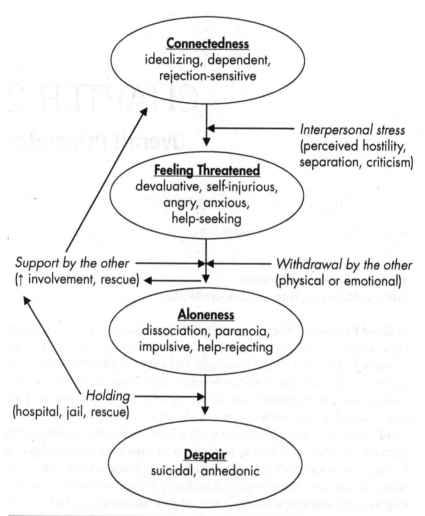

FIGURE 2–1.   Borderline personality disorder's interpersonal coherence.

Decreasing borderline patients' experiences of feeling threatened and alone does not usually depend on treaters. For borderline patients who live within stressful situations involving unexpected separations or hostility, their vacillating but basically negative sense of self remains unmodifiable. Some borderline patients will paradoxically cling to stressful relationships or situations, but helping those patients to attain more supportive and stable environments within which they can gain a more positive sense of self can be of substantial and enduring help.

Basic Therapeutic Approach

See Video 2, Diagnostic Disclosure
Video 3, Establishing an Alliance
Video 4, Managing Intersession Availability
Video 5, Managing Safety
Video 6, Managing Anger
Video 7, Managing Medications
Video 8, Managing Safety and Medications
Video 9, Managing Family Involvement

GPM holds that eight basic principles should guide treatment of BPD (see Table 2–1).

1. Offer Psychoeducation

It is helpful to share your knowledge about BPD and even your wisdom about life. Formal psychoeducation about BPD applies to every form of intervention, and examples of how to do this will be evident throughout this book. Informal psychoeducation involves reminding patients of their long-term goals (getting a life), and giving wise advice about romantic or vocational prospects, or even about more mundane things such as transportation and shopping.

2. Be Active, Not Reactive

Borderline patients need to know that you are present. Be responsive, don't accept silences, and raise questions if the patient does not show reactions to what is being said. Being quiet, passive, or minimizing their complaints is experienced as hostile or abandoning. However, do not overreact. Comments about suicide, violence, or other potential disasters require concerned examination. Overreacting with responses such as hospitalizations, medication changes, or consultations will be harmful.

3. Be Thoughtful

Being thoughtful, reflective, cautious, and uncertain are essential parts of containing ("holding") patients. Their world is black or white, all or nothing, and good or bad. Such dichotomous positions are rarely realistic. As explicated and emphasized in Mentalization-Based Treatment (Bateman and Fonagy 2012), you must be comfortable—even insistent—about "not knowing." Your comfort with being uncertain or undecided acts as a container for the patient's polarized black-or-white thinking and provides a model for his or her introjection. Being thoughtful does not mean that you do not need to be active, clear, directive, or authoritative.

TABLE 2–1.   **Basic principles of GPM**

Principle	Comment
1. Offer psychoeducation.	Don't hesitate to inform patients about what you know—or don't know—about their diagnosis and its treatment. Also, feel free to give advice when you feel it will be instructive.
2. Be active, not reactive.	Being responsive assures patients that you are interested and involved; do not catastrophize.
3. Be thoughtful.	You are a container for your patient's anxiety and a role model for "thinking first."
4. The relationship is real as well as professional.	Both aspects are necessary.
5. Convey that change is expected.	Its absence raises questions about the treatment's value.
6. Foster accountability.	Encourage being responsible for behavior, most notably for within-treatment failures to remember or implement the lessons learned in prior sessions.
7. Maintain a focus on life outside of treatment.	Stay informed about outside relationships, emphasize the value of structured vocational activities.
8. Be flexible, pragmatic, and eclectic.	Your responses and interventions are determined by the patient and good sense.

4. The Therapy Relationship Is Real (Dyadic) As Well As Professional

Acknowledge your mistakes (e.g., "I misunderstood," "I should have...," "If I could do it over, I'd..."). Fear of making mistakes can rob both you and the patient of an essential humanizing process (see also the principle "Change Is Expected" below). Accept idealization, but do not encourage unrealistic expectations ("I'm flattered that you think...," "My experience was different than you think..."). Self-disclosure can be helpful or harmful: do not deny the obvious or that the patient affects you, and always consider whether self-disclosure will help the patient (see Table 2–2).

5. Change Is Expected

Inform patients with BPD that the usual course of their disorder is one of gradual improvement. Underscore that whether improvement will occur depends

TABLE 2–2.	Self-disclosure by clinicians in treating borderline personality disorder

Anonymity is a myth—what varies is the accuracy of a patient's perceptions; we affect this.

Ways that self-disclosure can help:

- Normalizes feelings and beliefs that patients feel shamed by
- Encourages hope
- Establishes authenticity
- Gives permission to feel, say, act

on their taking on an active role. They can count on you to assist. Identify as long-term goals that they may be able to achieve satisfactory work and partnerships but that those also will depend on their efforts and chance.

6. Accountability

Hold patients responsible for what they say while retaining the leavening attitudes that your patient's mistakes, intolerance, hostility, or offensive behaviors are understandable and can change. Within sessions, remind patients of prior discussions; ask whether they had forgotten the conclusions reached, and, if they have, question how they could do that. Do not reflexively try to diminish guilt or shame; sometimes experiencing and acknowledging such feelings should be applauded. When these feelings can be borne without action or dissociation, they are preconditions and incentives for remorse, apologies, reconciliation, and change. The converse side of this is the clinician's need to be accountable for his or her own mistakes, feelings, or attitudes. Be ready to own these.

7. Focus on Life Outside of Treatment

Know what is happening in your patients' primary relationships and, given their instability, discuss the interpersonal perceptions and reactions as they recur. Most of their emotional (e.g., anger) and behavioral (e.g., self-harm) problems are related to interpersonal events. They need to recognize this. You can help them manage situational stressors. Sometimes wise advice is sufficient. Sometimes you should invite input from others (e.g., talks with members of the family). Interpersonal hypersensitivity can be buffered by having structured vocational activities. Clinicians should emphasize the message of "work before love" and encourage and aid vocational initiatives. Even by 6 months, borderline patients should be expected to have some school, work, or domestic responsibilities (see Table 2–3). Although a trusting and dependent relationship with you signals a positive development, the relationship can become an idealized substitute for real relationships. When this occurs, it signals an empty life, and consultation, and probably referral to a BPD specialist, is needed.

8. Be Flexible, Pragmatic, and Eclectic

To what extent you serve as coach, adviser, observer, or interpreter is determined by your patient. Borderline patients vary widely in their responsiveness to directions, criticisms, or interpretations: all can be helpful or harmful. The value of an intervention depends on the patient's current state of mind. Directives (or advice) are usually welcomed only after first asking whether your patient would like your opinion. As illustrated in Figure 2–1, emergency (high-stress) situations usually exacerbate defensiveness; more support is needed. Feeling "held" or connected increases acceptance of uninvited negative feedback (e.g., criticisms and interpretations). Similarly, management strategies for availability between sessions, missed sessions, or crises should be adapted to your patient rather than your policy (see sections "Intersession Availability" in Chapter 4 ["Getting Started" and "Impending Self-Endangering Behaviors" in Chapter 5 ["Managing Suicidality and Non-suicidal Self-Harm"]).

How Change Occurs

See Case 5, Lawrence, in Chapter 8 ("Case Illustrations")

The basic model of therapeutic action in GPM is that the treaters behave and respond in ways that are essentially distinct from prior relationships and that are corrective, in effect as well as intent, toward the BPD patient's interpersonal sensitivity. Within this model, Table 2–3 summarizes three processes by which change occurs with GPM.

Learning to "Think First"

Therapists should explicitly encourage patients to think before acting and reinforce this by complimenting them when they do this. Chain analyses, introspection, writing, talking, and "counting to 10" are all activities that therapists should urge to help patients delay acting on impulses. Learning to distrust initial reactions or to consider alternative perspectives are significant components of how mentalization-based treatment helps patients learn to think first. Accurate interpretations, best delivered as casual questions, can be very helpful (e.g., "I wonder whether that comment didn't make

TABLE 2–3.	GPM's therapeutic processes
Process	Comment
Learning to "think first"	This process involves learning to think before acting, being aware of and able to label feelings, and thinking about one's experience and those within others (identifying feelings and motives)—called *mentalizing*.
Social rehabilitation	This process includes learning to take initiative toward assuming social responsibilities (e.g., improve reliability, decrease procrastination, accept authority/ rules) or to chitchat with strangers, live within a budget, improve activities of daily living, and so on.
Corrective experiences	Being listened to, cared for, and given realistic expectations are new experiences that improve trust, self-disclosure, capacity for closeness, and humility. Therapists who are trusting, reasonable, and reliable model qualities that can be internalized.

you angry."). This learning process translates into borderline patients' deficient prefrontal cortex gaining control over their unruly amygdala (Donegan et al. 2003; Silbersweig et al. 2007).

Social Rehabilitation

As absorbing as the life crises and intense interpersonal interactions with borderline patients usually are, clinicians have to steadfastly keep an eye on their need to "get a life." Vocational stability is easier to attain than the exclusive relationship they believe they need. Patients will generally resist this redirection. If they attain satisfactory work and stable interpersonal support, their crises disappear, and their therapy becomes "obsolete."

Clinicians should explicitly identify the importance of attaining or resuming a social role or function. Much of patients' future happiness depends on finding strong and enduring partners and vocations. Those attainments then are self-perpetuating. Help patients recognize how their inexperience, unreliability, fears of failure, intolerance of criticism, difficulties asking for help, and so forth handicap attaining these goals. This is the *validation* part of one of Dialectical Behavior Therapy's basic dialectics. Then comes the *change* part. Encourage your patient to take on work or classes in which failure is least likely: volunteer before paid work; part-time before full-time work; easy class before hard class; familiar before unfamiliar. Underscore prior achievements, encourage "getting back on the horse," but be cautious of making "you can do it" statements—they are often heard as your minimizing the difficulty or blaming them for past failures.

Corrective Experiences

Being listened to ("heard") and being understood are often new or rare experiences for borderline patients. Reasonable expectations of being responsible for oneself and for one's future are often also new experiences. Trusting that you are truly and primarily invested in their welfare is often a new experience. You become a transitional object who silently confers security (Gunderson 1996). By being reliable, consistent, and responsible and by accepting authority, mistakes, and personal limitations, treaters model behaviors and attitudes that patients can introject with enduring benefits. Those within-treatment corrective experiences set the stage for patients becoming more likely to find stable partners or jobs, which become their own corrective experiences.

CHAPTER 3
Making the Diagnosis

Disclosure of the Diagnosis

See Video 1, Psychoeducation
See also Case 1, Roger, in Chapter 8 ("Case Illustrations")

Most borderline patients initially seek help for another problem (e.g., depression, somatic complaints, self-harm, substance abuse, insomnia). The diagnosis of borderline personality disorder (BPD) may then become evident only through the issues that arise after clinicians begin treating these presenting problems (e.g., your patient distrusts your motives, tests your availability, misuses prescriptions, or becomes unexpectedly angry). After the borderline diagnosis has become evident, many clinicians still remain hesitant to disclose the diagnosis (see Table 3–1). Yet there are significant reasons why giving patients this diagnosis is of definite clinical value (see Table 3–1).

The Diagnosis Anchors the Patient's and the Clinician's Expectations About Course

Even when priority must be given to symptoms, behaviors, or situational crises, the added perspective derived from the BPD diagnosis is that the patient has long-term serious handicaps. For those BPD patients who present with depression, anxiety, eating disorders, or substance abuse, the diagnosis of BPD yields knowledge about which diagnoses should be the primary target and what can and cannot be expected from medications (see Chapter 6 ["Pharmacotherapy and Comorbidity"]).

TABLE 3–1.   **Disclosure of the borderline personality disorder (BPD) diagnosis**

Why clinicians do not disclose the diagnosis:

• I can help this patient without making the diagnosis (sometimes true, often not).

• The patient will feel ashamed or criticized (a countertransference projection).

• I don't believe I can treat BPD.

Why clinicians should disclose the diagnosis:

• Establishes realistic expectations about course and treatment

• Facilitates a treatment alliance

• Prepares the treater: beware of one's countertransference

The Borderline Diagnosis Establishes a Basis for Developing a Treatment Alliance

The BPD diagnosis offers patients and their families a developmental and therapeutic context that they will experience as meaningful and appropriate. As described later in this chapter, an alliance is facilitated by the initial reassurance that borderline patients feel upon learning that their problems are shared by others, that treatment can help, and that their treaters have a body of relevant knowledge to draw from. Table 3–2 summarizes knowledge that patients and families should attain.

The Diagnosis Prepares Clinicians for What's Ahead

The borderline diagnosis should increase your awareness of the patient's interpersonal sensitivity and his or her potential to accept (idealize) or reject (devalue) your help unthinkingly. Without realizing the borderline diagnosis, you might respond to these reactions with caregiving or anger, respectively, whereas knowing the diagnosis should yield a more helpful response, such as curiosity. Indeed, it was because interventions that for most nonborderline patients are helpful (e.g., support without contingencies, disapproval without apologies) seemed to make borderline patients worse, that the need arose to identify the particular signs and symptoms of what we now call "borderline" (Gunderson 2009). Clinicians who understand the borderline patient's typical hypersensitivity to caregivers and who, as a result, adjust their caregiving find that they can be far more helpful than they expected. Unfortunately, when clinicians are unaware that their patient has the BPD diagnosis, their naïve responses can aggravate their patients' problems and can impel them to reject or be rejected by their patients.

TABLE 3–2.	Basic psychoeducation: what every borderline patient and his or her family should know

- **Borderline personality disorder (BPD) is significantly heritable** (~55%). This means that families need to customize their caregiving to accommodate the handicaps due to the borderline family member's genetic disposition.

- **BPD is a disorder that is very sensitive to environmental stress,** especially interpersonal stressors (anger, rejection) or the lack of structure (inconsistent, unpredictable, ambiguous). This means that patients get relief from structured and supportive environments. Neurobiological correlates involve elevated cortisol levels and opioid deficits.

- **The brains of people with BPD have a hyperreactive amygdala** (easily excited) **and an underactive prefrontal cortex** (less cognitive/thinking inhibitions). Almost all effective therapies enhance prefrontal cortical activity, imposing thinking to evaluate perceptions and to control behaviors and feelings.

- **Most patients with BPD have symptom remissions** (about 50% by 2 years, 85% by 10 years), and once remitted, only about 15% relapse. However, their symptom improvement is associated with only modest improvements in social adaptation (i.e., only about one-third achieve stable marriages or full-time employment by 10 years).

- **There are multiple forms of empirically validated treatment for BPD.** All decrease self-harm, anger, and depression and use of hospitals, emergency departments, and medications. These treatments usually require 1–3 hours per week for a year or more by therapists with extensive training and ongoing supervision.

- **The vast majority of BPD patients improve very significantly without receiving these therapies.** Good Psychiatric Management is usually sufficient. Treatment with intensive BPD-specific therapies should be sought for patients who do not respond.

How to Disclose

See Video 2, Diagnostic Disclosure

The following form of disclosure involves the developmental perspective that was illustrated in Figure 2–1 (see Chapter 2 ["Overall Principles"]):

> "People with BPD are born with a genetic disposition to be highly sensitive and reactive to their caretakers. They are more apt to attribute rejection or anger to parental behaviors than are other children. They have usually grown up feeling that they were unfairly treated and that they did not get the attention or care they needed. They resent this and, as young adults, they hope to

establish a relationship with someone who can make up to them for what they feel is missing. The desired relationship is exclusive, setting in motion intense reactions to real or perceived slights, rejections, or separations. Predictably, both their unrealistic expectations and their intense reactions cause such relationships to fail. When this happens, people with BPD will feel rejected or abandoned, and they cannot resolve their anger about being treated unfairly and their fear that they are bad and deserved the rejection. Both conclusions can lead them to become self-destructive. Their anger about being mistreated or their shame about being bad or their self-destructive behaviors can evoke guilty or protective feelings in others. Such guilt or rescuing responses from others validate the borderline person's unrealistically negative perceptions of mistreatment and sustain their unrealistically high expectations of having their needs met. Thus, the cycle is apt to repeat itself."

An easier and less theoretical way to disclose the borderline diagnosis is to invite the patient to review the criteria and let you know if they "fit." This process involves the patient in making his or her own diagnosis and is, in itself, alliance building.

Common Problems

Your Patient Refuses the Borderline Diagnosis

Patients may refuse the borderline diagnosis when they think the diagnosis blames them for their problems, when they have heard it used pejoratively about other patients, or when the diagnosis challenges preexisting diagnoses from cherished prior treaters. In any case, your patient does not need to accept the diagnosis per se. What is important is to identify some more discrete treatment goals the patient can accept. For example, "Let's see whether medications will help with your [anxiety/depression, etc.]" or "Let's try to change your ex-husband's views about his alcohol abuse." If you work on these issues successfully, the goals can shift toward other more BPD-specific issues (e.g., sense of badness, episodic rages, rejection sensitivity) without the BPD diagnosis needing to be accepted. Still, it will be useful to eventually re-present the BPD diagnosis for the reasons identified earlier.

You Believe Your Patient Has Borderline Personality Disorder, But She or He Does Not Meet the DSM Threshold

The DSM diagnostic algorithm is not set in stone. The interpersonal criteria are most central (e.g., splits in self-image or in perceptions of others, abandonment fears, fears of aloneness, excessive rejection sensitivity) (Gunderson and Lyons-Ruth 2008). In addition, other signature criteria include excessive anger and self-destructive behaviors (Grilo et al. 2007). The presence of any three of these should make it difficult to not diagnose BPD. In the absence of at least three of these, another diagnosis might be more useful.

CHAPTER 4
Getting Started

Setting the Framework

See Video 3, Establishing an Alliance

> "I'd be glad to meet with you weekly, but whether we should meet more often and for how long are questions that depend on whether I can be useful. We'll both know that by observing whether you feel better and whether these problems in your behavior, such as anger and self-harm, and in your relationships, such as distrust and possessiveness, diminish."

Good Psychiatric Management (GPM) usually involves once-weekly visits with uncertain expectations about their duration (Table 4–1)—the idea being that the duration (and frequency) will be determined by whether the patient is finding the visits useful. Adding more frequent sessions can then follow a patient's inclination, with the caveat that clinicians should not initiate a schedule of more than twice a week without either considerable prior experience or supervision. When the primary clinician is a psychiatrist, his or her role will usually include medication management, perhaps using a consultant for complicated questions (see Chapter 6 ["Pharmacotherapy and Comorbidity"]). When feasible, borderline patients should be encouraged to participate in another form of treatment (e.g., group, family therapy, or self-help groups; see Chapter 7 ["Split Treatments"]). All providers should have access to and readiness to use consultation. When the patient participates in more than one form of treatment, he or she should understand that the treaters will speak to one another as they deem necessary (see Case 1, Roger, in Chapter 8 ["Case Illustrations"]).

TABLE 4–1.   **GPM's framework**

- Sessions are held once weekly.

- Duration depends on progress.

- Adjunctive (split) treatments (group, family, medication) are desirable.

- Consultations and peer discussions are desirable.

Assessing Progress

You should encourage patients to assess whether this treatment is helpful but retain an independent responsibility for monitoring and discussing whether change is occurring. Changes occur sequentially: improvements in subjective distress can be expected at about 1–3 weeks, in behavior at 2–6 months, in interpersonal relationships at 6–12 months, and in social adaptation (i.e., "getting a life") at 6–18 months (see Table 4–2).

You should use introspection to assess change as well: 1) Do I understand the patient better? 2) Can I now predict my patient's reactions (e.g., what prompts anger or self-harm)? 3) Am I involved (e.g., Do I worry/think about the patient between sessions)? and 4) Has the patient become more trusting, more able to depend on me? Failure to observe these changes should raise questions about whether you are useful to the patient.

Do not hesitate to explicitly raise the question of whether a treatment is useful, especially in the early stages of treatment (see Case 5, Lawrence, in Chapter 8). Table 4–3 offers change makers—based on usual expectable progress—that should prompt this question. There are many exceptions. However, if you and your patient cannot find some reassuring answers to the question of effectiveness, it is time to seek consultation.

Intersession Availability

See Video 4, Managing Intersession Availability

> "Should an emergency arise, I would like to be helpful. More generally, I would like you to grow confident about my concern for your welfare. However, since you cannot count on my always being available, we should discuss alternative plans. What do you propose?"

It is best to start with the assumption that your patient has managed and can continue to manage personal crises between scheduled sessions (see Gunderson 1996; Nadort et al. 2009). Only when this is clearly not true or the patient asks about your availability should the issue be addressed. Your

TABLE 4–2.   **Sequence of expectable changes**

Target area	Changes	Time	Relevant interventions
Subjective distress or dysphoria	↓ Anxiety and depression	1–3 weeks	Support, situational changes ↑ Self-awareness
Behavior	↓ Self-harm, rages, and promiscuity	2–6 months	↑ Awareness of self and interpersonal triggers ↑ Problem-solving strategies
Interpersonal relationships	↓ Devaluation ↑ Assertiveness + Dependency[a]	6–12 months	↑ Mentalization ↑ Stability of attachment
Social function	School/work/ domestic responsibilities	6–18 months	↓ Fear, failure, and abandonment; coaching

[a]A positive and dependent relationship to the therapist has formed.

Source.   Adapted from Gunderson JG, Links P: *Borderline Personality Disorder: A Clinical Guide,* 2nd Edition. Washington, DC, American Psychiatric Publishing, 2008. Used with permission.

response should keep the patient responsible for his or her own welfare as much as possible (see "Accountability" subsection in Chapter 2 ["Overall Principles"]).

Figure 4–1 outlines a strategy for managing intersession availability. If your patient does not call on you during crises, discuss what that means: does he or she think that you would not want to be called, that you don't care, or that it wouldn't be helpful? If the patient did call and it did not seem like a crisis, the next session offers an excellent opportunity to increase your patient's awareness of core fears of aloneness, being uncared for, and using others as transitional objects. In the unusual circumstance when limits need to be set, do so by saying, "I'm sorry, but responding to your calls has become too difficult for me. Let's consider what other ways you can get support."

Cyberspace has created new options for communication. Electronic messages (e-mail, Facebook, text messaging) are useful for appointment changes and can be a vehicle for conveying homework. The fantasy of being in communication can be a form of transitional relatedness that can be calming. Treaters should clarify, however, that this is not a reliable way to communicate anything urgent and not usually a feasible way to communicate anything very lengthy. Treaters also should inform patients that their messages will be discussed in the following session.

TABLE 4–3.   **When to question whether treatment is failing**

Time in treatment	Observation
3 weeks	Attendance is poor.
	Subjective distress is not better.
	You do not like the patient.
3 months	Patient consistently disparages the therapy.
	Self-endangering events or activities of daily living (e.g., sleep, diet) worsen.
	Your empathy or understanding has not improved.
6 months	Level of self-endangering behaviors persists.
	Patient fails to remember or use lessons from prior sessions.
	Patient has failed to attain or resume some part-time vocational role.
	Patient fails to recognize significance of adverse interpersonal events such as rejection or separations.

The expectation that treating patients with BPD requires being available 24/7 for recurrent emergencies, usually involving a possible suicide attempt, is rarely justified. Clinicians encourage this idea by inviting calls without crises, by offering prolonged supportive listening on receipt of calls, and by not following up on intersession contacts by examining their necessity, their value, and possible alternatives. Any borderline patient who insists that 24/7 availability is necessary should be referred to BPD specialists—who, by using either a team or a residential setting, can make such availability feasible.

Building an Alliance

See Video 3, **Establishing an Alliance**
Video 7, **Managing Medications**
Video 9, **Managing Family Involvement**

The basic therapeutic stance of concerned attention, steadfast listening, and validation for the patients' painful experiences are necessities on which the various forms of alliance are built. Showing trust in your good intentions

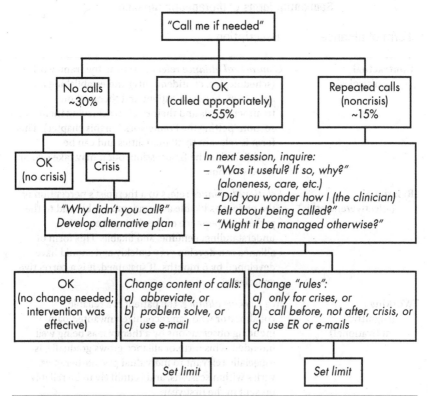

FIGURE 4–1. Algorithm for intersession availability of therapist.
ER = emergency room.

and a willingness to follow your advice are signs of an alliance that represents achievements for borderline patients—these are not preconditions for treating BPD. Table 4–4 identifies the sequence in which the different forms of a therapeutic alliance are established.

The following interventions facilitate alliance building; they all act to engage patients in collaborating with you toward their improvement.

Psychoeducation

Psychoeducation establishes parameters for hopefulness, affirms the necessity of patients' participation, and acquaints them with the knowledge base from which your clinical judgments derive (see "Offer Psychoeducation" subsection in Chapter 2). Encouraging them to read about the disorder and its treatment is a good first step toward this end. Suggest books or Internet sites (see Gunderson and Links 2008 for a guide).

TABLE 4–4.   **Sequential forms of therapeutic alliance**

Form of alliance	Description
Contractual (goals/roles)	*Contractual alliance* refers to setting the framework (schedule, fee, confidentiality) and establishing an agreement between patient and therapist on treatment goals and their roles in achieving them (see section "Setting the Framework" in this chapter). This form is relevant to all modalities and can be established in the first session, but it may take two or three sessions.
Relational (affective/empathic)	*Relational alliance* refers to a therapist's perception of the patient as likable and understandable and to the patient's experience of the therapist as caring, understanding, genuine, and likable. This form of alliance can develop very quickly and should have developed by 6 months. If sustained, it is a corrective experience.
Working (cognitive/ motivational)	In a *working alliance,* the patient is a reliable collaborator who can recognize unwanted pain-inducing observations by a therapist as being well intended. This form of alliance grows gradually, is especially relevant to individual psychotherapies, varies within sessions, and is unlikely to be reliably present in the first year.

Medications

Prescribing medications to relieve borderline patients' characteristically severe level of subjective distress (Zanarini et al. 1998) usually expedites their perception of your good will (see Chapter 6).

Homework

Asking patients to work on their self-understanding and therapy issues between sessions underscores their need to think and to be active participants. Tell patients that in-session talks are insufficient—they need to continue giving attention to their issues after they leave the office. Making reference to thoughts that you have had about them or to prior sessions encourages this and encourages your transitional object role. Homework can take many forms.

Write an autobiography. This is a great way to build a narrative, but patients may resist or find it difficult. Simplify by asking patients to start with major events or a family tree, then make fleshing it out a process that is returned to. Enlist their involvement with specific questions if you write out a life chart.

Detail a recent crisis. What is called *chain analysis* is an important process quite aside from the content or the insights gained. It underscores cause and effect through discussion within sessions and then becomes progressively more detailed in highlighting how a sequential thought, feeling, and action process might have been intercepted, if recognized, before the crisis.

Fill out structured forms. This activity can involve any type of self-assessment (e.g., personality questionnaires, mood monitors, computerized research instruments). Filling out safety plans (see Chapter 5 ["Managing Suicidality and Nonsuicidal Self-Harm"] and Video 5, Managing Safety) or charting the rise or fall of target symptoms in response to medications (see Chapter 6 and Video 8, Managing Safety and Medications) are good forms of homework. In the future patients may use applications on their smartphones or other mobile devices to rate their experiences as they are happening. These ratings can automatically be sent to their therapists.

Setting Goals

The initial goals should be short-term and feasible (e.g., leaving a stressful situation, calling for support, improving sleep, attending a self-help group). Although such agreed-on goals are helpful, borderline patients in crises, with little sense of identity, with alexithymia, or with profound distrust, may be unable to do this meaningfully. For them, establishing goals is a goal in itself and a process within the treatment.

Other Interventions

These other interventions facilitate alliance building:

- Active pursuit or calling about missed appointments (see Case 5, Lawrence, in Chapter 8)
- Coaching about situations (see "Offer Psychoeducation" subsection in Chapter 2)
- Doing for a patient what the patient says he or she cannot do (e.g., help set up an appointment with a nutritionist); this must be done with discretion (see Gunderson 2007)

Common Problems

Changing Therapists

Problems arise when you, acting as an inpatient director of care or a consultant, conclude that an existing therapy is ineffective or harmful, but either the treater or the patient does not agree. This reaction may occur because the judgment of ineffectiveness or harm has been personalized (i.e., it is experienced as an assault on the therapist's competence or character). A way to depersonalize your recommendation for change when discussing it with another treater is to explain it in terms of the lack of expected improvement in subjective distress, self-harm, and suicidality and use of emergency department and hospital facilities (see section "Basic Therapeutic Approach" in Chapter 2). Note that a change to a different treater is usual, not rare. If it is solely the patient who is resisting a change of treater (or treatment), this may reflect a reaction to the proposed separation. When this is the case, you can encourage a follow-up meeting in, say, 3 months with the previous treater or establish a plan for that therapy to resume when specified changes (e.g., stop cutting, be gainfully employed) have occurred. It is often sufficient to request the prior therapist's explicit support for the change or, if necessary, encourage that therapist to set limits on his or her ongoing availability. If both the treater and the patient resist change, you may need to be content with documenting your opinion and advising the treater to obtain consultation or ongoing supervision.

Patient Refuses to Accept the Framework

The framework should initially be flexible (see sections "Basic Therapeutic Approach" in Chapter 2 and "Setting the Framework" earlier in this chapter). Patients' refusals to let you talk with prior treaters or family members, to discuss or agree upon goals, to seek help when suicidal, or to stop drinking exemplify issues that greatly handicap the likelihood that treatment will succeed. Still, these should be considered obstacles that might change if the patient develops an alliance. Only after you have concluded that such resistances are incompatible with the patient's safety or with your ability to be helpful should treatment be suspended. In contrast, other refusals may be incompatible with treatment of the BPD condition, such as persistent intoxication, nonattendance, nonpayment, or for patients in serious danger, their refusal to adopt any reasonable safety plan (see section "Common Problems" in Chapter 5).

Patient Cannot Relate to, Feel Connected to, or Become Attached to Treater

You may judge that the patient's lack of connection to the treater is defensive or part of a broader "help-rejecting" agenda, but do not challenge it. When being "disconnected" is a form of dissociation, the patient could benefit from psychoeducation (*"This is a symptom of extensive stress, usually intermittent, that will diminish when you develop stable attachments"*) or from grounding exercises. Within psychotherapies, persistently feeling disconnected for six to eight sessions should stimulate a referral. Help the patient find someone he or she might connect with, but don't be surprised if the patient returns.

You Don't Like Your Patient

Not liking your patient will be a serious impediment to being helpful. After a few sessions, however, backing out can be difficult if the patient does not reciprocate this feeling. If the reasons for the dislike will make any therapy unlikely (patient's hygiene, dismissiveness, disrespect, or silence), this should be discussed and the patient given an opportunity to change. If the dislike is a result of your personal aversions (e.g., appearance, politics, dependency, hostility), these (as "countertransference issues") should be discussed with a colleague or therapist. If they are beyond your ability to change, consider—with due apologies—telling the patient that you consider yourself a bad match because of *your* limitations and that she or he deserves to work with someone more apt to be compatible.

You Will Be Unavailable for an Extended Time

The same principles described earlier (see section "Building an Alliance") apply. As much as possible, keep the patient responsible for planning any treatment contacts. Making yourself available by telephone or e-mail is fine if you know it will not interfere with your plans. Coverage should be arranged if the patient wants it—even though the patient may not use it (see Case 4, Laura, in Chapter 8).

CHAPTER 5

Managing Suicidality and Nonsuicidal Self-Harm

Recurrent suicidal acts, threats, impulses, or the perception of their likelihood is the "signature" symptom of borderline personality disorder (BPD) that usually precipitates the diagnosis (see Table 5–1). The risk, even the probability, of having a BPD patient attempt suicide is inherent in taking on many of these cases. This aspect of BPD creates the most anxiety about personal competence and the most fear of liability in treaters. Although suicidal ideas and self-destructive actions are usually recurrent, clinicians should appreciate that this is one of the first areas in which behavioral improvement is usually discernible. As noted in Figure 2–1 in Chapter 2 ("Overall Principles"), this usually signals that the patient believes that you (or someone) cares or that he or she is engaged in a treatment that can help. As has also been noted (see sections "Basic Therapeutic Approach" and "How Change Occurs" in Chapter 2 and subsection "Assessing Progress" in Chapter 4 ["Getting Started"]; see also Case 4, Laura, in Chapter 8 ["Case Illustrations"]), failure to improve in this area should raise questions about the treatment's utility.

A treater's sense of burden and risk of liability, the patient's course, and the associated health care costs are all intimately connected with how self-endangering behaviors are managed. Table 5–2 clarifies liability concerns—they are truly minimal if you discuss your patient's safety or other treatment issues with others.

37

TABLE 5–1.	Borderline personality disorder's "behavioral specialty": suicidality and self-harm

- The risk of suicide is significant—estimates vary from 3% to 10%.
    - This rate is particularly high within the young female demographic.

- About 75% self-harm; among these, 90% do so repeatedly.
    - Self-harm increases the risk of suicide 15–30 times.

- Suicidal acts are ambivalent (e.g., If rescued, I want to live. If not, I prefer to die.)
    - The average number of suicide attempts is 3.
    - Suicide occurs once per 23 attempts.

- Suicidal and self-harm acts are often preceded by interpersonal stress, substance abuse, and increasing depression.

- Outpatient therapy significantly reduces the risk of suicide and self-harm.

Source.   Links and Kolla 2005; Stanley et al. 2001; Yen et al. 2004, 2005, 2009.

Impending Self-Endangering Behaviors

See Video 5, Managing Safety
See also section "Basic Therapeutic Approach" in Chapter 2

"Suicidality and self-endangering behaviors are usually reactions to interpersonal stress.[1] I can help you to manage these situations, but to diminish their cause, we need to help you get a better social support network—people to help you with those situations."

The general principle is that *clinicians should always respond to even indirect communications of self-endangering behaviors with concern, but assessing the patient's actual dangerousness is essential.* The corollaries of this principle are described in the following subsections.

Assess Suicidality and Dangerousness

While expressing concern, do not suspend your need to make a careful clinical judgment about the actual dangerousness. This involves assessing recent losses (including diminished treatment) and increased depression or substance use (see Figure 5–1).

---

[1] I.e., the perception of rejection and the fear of being alone; see Figure 2–1.

TABLE 5–2.	Liability concerns in treating self-endangering behaviors in borderline patients

- The risk of liability is higher than for most psychiatric patients but remains low (<1%) and becomes negligible among experienced clinicians.

- Liability largely derives from countertransference enactments—excessive availability, punitive hostility, personal involvement, and illusions of omniscience or omnipotence.

- Liability can be minimized by discussing your patients with colleagues, by using consultants, or by having split treatments.

The most critical issue is differentiating suicidal from nonsuicidal intentions. Too often, cutting oneself is assumed to be suicidal. Often it is a deliberate act that is self-soothing or self-punitive or a cry for help. Concluding that the actual risk is low or that the patient's intention is manipulative (a "call for help" or a wish to invoke guilt) can decrease hospitalizations and limit secondary gain. However, if such conclusions get expressed by a clinician's hostility or dismissiveness, recurrence of suicidality or self-harm, now with increased dangerousness, becomes likely. Clinicians who exaggerate the risk may insist on ritualized and excessive suicide evaluations that reinforce the use of suicide threats to solicit help. To avoid this problem, the clinician and patient should discuss the need to differentiate nonlethal self-harm behavior from "true" suicidal intention.

A valuable strategy is to ask your patient to develop a personal method of rating his or her level of emotional distress and risk of suicide. The scale also should identify the appropriate individuals to contact along the continuum of perceived self-harm risk levels from safe to unsafe. This provides patients with a tool to communicate better with their support network about their needs. The clinician should help the patient develop the scale and then follow up with revisions or expansions as the patient learns to understand himself or herself better. Moving beyond an inherent dichotomous all-or-nothing thinking, this practice reinforces the thinking-before-acting principle (see subsection "Learning to 'Think First'" in Chapter 2).

Select the Appropriate Level of Care

Selecting the appropriate level of care (Figure 5–2; see also Case 4, Laura, in Chapter 8) follows from the assessment of dangerousness. Fortunately, outpatient services are usually sufficient for borderline patients after the evaluating clinicians have carefully weighed the potential risk of using this lower level of care against the potential harm from using a higher level of care. Unfortunately, clinicians reflexively often seek higher levels of care to

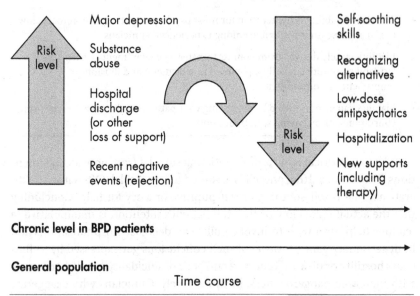

Acute exacerbation of risk

Risk level (upward arrow):
- Major depression
- Substance abuse
- Hospital discharge (or other loss of support)
- Recent negative events (rejection)

Risk level (downward arrow):
- Self-soothing skills
- Recognizing alternatives
- Low-dose antipsychotics
- Hospitalization
- New supports (including therapy)

Chronic level in BPD patients

General population

Time course

FIGURE 5–1.   Acute-on-chronic suicide risk.

In patients with borderline personality disorder (BPD), the acute-on-chronic level of suicide risk (***curved arrow***) can change more quickly than in the general population and will be modified by several factors that can cause (***upward arrow***) and several that might reduce (***downward arrow***) an acute exacerbation of risk.

Source.   Adapted from Gunderson JG, Links P: *Borderline Personality Disorder: A Clinical Guide,* 2nd Edition. Washington, DC, American Psychiatric Publishing, 2008. Used with permission.

diminish their own anxiety. Moreover, many health care systems lack the intensive outpatient or residential levels of care, thereby forcing clinicians to use hospitals to manage self-endangering behaviors.

Invite the Patient to Tell You How You Might Help

See "Basic Therapeutic Approach," subsections "Be Active, Not Reactive" and "Change is Expected," in Chapter 2

Asking a patient to tell you how you can help underscores the patient's need to be active on his or her own behalf (reinforcing the sense of agency and the need to think) and discourages the use of suicidal or self-harm threats as a way to escape, avoid, or externalize responsibility. Do not expect patients to welcome this request; they may refuse or be unable to give meaningful

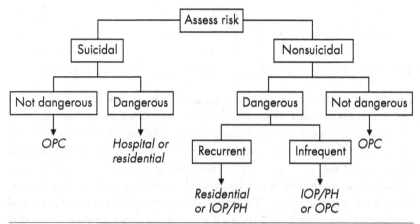

FIGURE 5–2.   Algorithm for selecting the level of care in response to self-endangering behaviors.

Levels of care:

1. OPC = outpatient clinic/office practice.
2. IOP/PH = intensive outpatient (>3 hours/week)/partial hospital (>10 hours/week).
3. Residential = structured living environments (e.g., halfway house).
4. Hospital.

answers. No matter. Simply note that your ability to help them is compromised by the absence of their input.

Be Clear About Your Limits

You are not omniscient, clairvoyant, or omnipotent. As noted in Chapter 4 (see section "Intersession Availability"), it is unrealistic for a patient's safety to depend on your availability. Tell the patient that you cannot be expected to know about his or her suicidality or self-harm unless the patient tells you. Even when you know about it, you may not be able to help the patient prevent it, and when such behaviors have already occurred, you may not be able to repair the damaging effects. "So, what use are you?" may be the response. Simply apologize for your limits.

Involve Colleagues

Involvement of colleagues is very important! Assessing and managing self-endangering behaviors is stressful and difficult. Ease your burden, minimize your liability, and diminish the risk of making harmful responses by discussing these issues with colleagues.

The Aftermath of Self-Endangering Behaviors

For Self-Harm or Unsuccessful Suicide Attempts

Identify in detail the chain of events and feelings that precipitated the self-endangering behavior. Do not accept the answer that nothing has occurred (i.e., a mood changed without any stressful event). That might be true for patients with a mood disorder but is not true for those with BPD. When patients do not volunteer accounts of rejection or aloneness, actively inquire about such events within their interpersonal relationships and most especially with you or other treaters. Asking patients to write this out in detail is a useful way to start this process. This review is essential for understanding (increasing self-awareness, accepting the impact of others), developing a sense of agency, and preventing recurrences. After an attempt, the patient's personal safety plan should be revisited and adapted based on the learning from this event.

Actively underscore the interpersonal context that both prompts and relieves self-endangering behaviors. Precipitants often involve the experiences of rejection or of being alone and being "bad." Relief involves the nonspecific experiences or perceptions of being cared for ("held") (see Figure 2–1 in Chapter 2). Such relief can come quietly via your clarification, questioning, or interpretation. It is very helpful for patients to accept the significance of their interpersonal sensitivity. The fact that you (or someone else) can understand this about them helps them feel less alone and less bad.

Anticipate future safety issues. Look ahead to future safety issues and develop a safety plan about alternative behaviors or ways to prevent recurrence. Have this discussion within the context of scheduled appointments when self-harm or suicidal behaviors have been repetitious or have been used for seeking help. This includes their effect on you (e.g., "It troubled me," "I had difficulty sleeping," "I wondered whether I had failed"). Identify the unfeasibility of depending on your availability and generate alternative ways of coping (e.g., distraction, seeking company, hotlines). Then proactively involve the patient in generating a plan to manage escalating levels of dangerousness (e.g., from impulse to planning) with a relevant set of actions (e.g., from meditation to calling 911) (see Appendix C, "Safety Planning: An Example" and Video 5, Managing Safety).

For Completed Suicides

Completed suicide by BPD patients usually involves questions (what if; if only…) about whether it could have been prevented. These questions reflect the ambivalence behind the borderline patients' attempts; usually, attempts are made under circumstances when others might have been expected to prevent them—their lives would have been made worth living if only someone had been there to rescue them.

Inform and document. Inform the authorities (hospital, police) and document your most recent interactions with the patient.

Discuss your reactions with colleagues, friends, and others. It is often very useful to recognize the precariousness of the patient's life in the absence of exclusive relationships.

Inform, offer solace, and encourage discussions with families. Interacting with the family is usually difficult because of your own feelings, but it is critically important for the family members.

Realize that this goes with the territory. Remind yourself that assuming responsibility for patients who might commit suicide was a cornerstone of your professional training.

Be forgiving, but learn. Have a "postmortem" conference to facilitate gaining perspective and learning (considerations of "could haves" and "should haves").

Common Problems

Your Patient's Suicidality Is Not Diminishing

If a patient's suicidal acts recur frequently (e.g., more than once every 3 months) or suicidality persists (e.g., fails to improve by 6 months), you should openly question whether the treatment is useful and, unless improvement is otherwise evident, insist on a more intensive multimodal treatment or refer the patient for more BPD-specific therapy or clinical service. If the patient refuses to participate, seek consultation (for you). In any event, look for ways that you might be unwittingly reinforcing (e.g., giving more attention during crises) or even stimulating (e.g., being too nurturant or too distant) the patient's suicidality. Dialectical behavior therapists sometimes ask patients to "take suicide off the table" (i.e., suspend that option for a period of weeks or months) as a condition for receiving Dialectical Behavior Therapy. This can be very effective for those patients who place a high value on receiving treatment from you, either because they believe you offer "something" distinctive or because they do not have any equivalent options.

The Patient Seeks Hospitalization for Suicidality, but You Do Not Think He or She Is Suicidal

If your patient will not give any assurance of "being safe" and you refuse to hospitalize him or her, the risk of a suicidal event is escalated. You think that hospitalization will reinforce a maladaptive pattern—and may irritate your colleagues within the hospital. (The same dilemma surrounds patients who insist on being medicated for self-endangering behaviors; see section "Common Problems" in Chapter 6 ["Pharmacotherapy and Comorbidity"].) Tell the patient:

> "I'm willing to hospitalize you despite my concern that it will not be helpful.
> I will do this because I fear you will become more suicidal if I don't. Am I
> right about that? We would both be better off if we could find an alternative."

This "false submission" takes the "magic" out of being hospitalized and calls on your patient to discuss why he or she might prefer being there—that is, because it means you really care (are "adopting" the patient) or because he or she covets being cared for without responsibilities. Having this discussion with your patient also helps disarm your emergency department or hospital staff colleagues who would otherwise be justifiably critical of your judgment.

Your Patient With Dangerous Suicidal or Self-Harming Behaviors Refuses to Give You Permission to Contact Significant Others

Even when the patient denies suicidal intentions but has recently been suicidal, you retain the legal right to make clinically indicated calls. When the patient's behaviors involve serious danger to self or if the self-endangering behaviors are related to interpersonal stress with significant others (e.g., therapists, family, spouse, roommates), it is a serious mistake not to insist on contacting these people. When a patient's suicidal behaviors have led to hospitalization, the hospital staff have responsibility to contact the patient's significant others. The patient's protestations that he or she is no longer suicidal, even if true, should not override the clinician's recognition that the risk of recurrent suicidal behaviors remains high. Even when the dangerousness is not serious, contacting the patient's significant others is an important part of suicide prevention and aftercare management.

Most suicidal or self-harm behaviors of borderline patients occur in a context of interpersonal stress. Involving the people who have evoked such reactions will facilitate talking through such events and, via psychoeducation, help those others become allies in the patient's treatment. A clinician's willingness to go along with a borderline patient's refusal to allow such involvement is most dangerous when the patient cohabits with or is financially dependent on those who are being kept uninformed. Failure to involve these people invites the patient to idealize you as a rescuer or to dismiss you as a weak link, someone needing these individuals' approval and avoiding their anger.

Your Patient Will Not Agree to Take Suicide "Off the Table"

For some very few borderline patients, the clinician needs to accept the possibility that they may kill themselves. For those patients, retaining this option is necessary; they retain a needed sense of control, or they cannot forgo this option because their future seems so desolate (Maltsberger et al. 2011). Clinicians who choose to work with such patients must ensure that they will not be liable in case of suicide (see Table 5–2). This involves two precautions: making sure that the patient's significant others understand and accept that suicide might occur, and consulting with another psychiatrist who confirms that other treatment options would not be safer.

Your Patient Will Not Agree to Decrease Self-Harm Behaviors

When the self-harm behaviors endanger the patient's health, cautions about potential liability (see Table 5–2) are warranted. Most of the time, the borderline patient's self-harm behaviors do not carry immediate or serious health issues and do not need to be a primary target of treatment. Clinicians can learn to appreciate the useful function such self-harm behaviors have for that patient. This understanding yields strategies that can help the patient decide to discontinue them; for example, if the self-harm is based on shame, expose the source(s); if the self-harm is based on self-hatred ("badness"), help the patient identify and accept his or her anger or hostility; and if the self-harm is generated by fear of rejection, being understood lessens that fear.

CHAPTER 6

Pharmacotherapy and Comorbidity

General Principles

Be Active, Not Reactive

See Video 1, Psychoeducation
Video 3, Establishing an Alliance
See also "Basic Therapeutic Approach," in Chapter 2 ("Overall Principles")

Good pharmacotherapeutic practices provide an important "holding" (containing) function for borderline patients. The practices described below reflect the basic principle that the relationship with the prescriber may be more valuable than the medications prescribed.

- If the patient requests medications but is not severely distressed, be willing but cautious and use selective serotonin reuptake inhibitors (SSRIs; they can have modest benefits and may help establish an alliance).
- If the patient is severely distressed but does not want medications, encourage their use if you think that will decrease distress, but even then, do not push.
- Establish a policy that if the patient is failing to respond to a medication, you will taper it and only then begin another medication (unless the patient is severely distressed, in which case you should cross taper).
- Acutely distressed patients need to learn self-soothing; initiating new medications may have placebo effects but otherwise can have only limited expectable benefits.

47

Avoid a Dichotomous Stance

You should avoid a dichotomous stance—that is, assertion that medications either will or will not be helpful and either will or will not be harmful. Convey uncertainty and caution, offer measured hope, and encourage thinking (increase prefrontal cortical activity).

Building an Alliance

See Video 7, Managing Medications
Video 8, Managing Safety and Medications
See also Chapter 3 ("Making the Diagnosis")

> "I'd like you to try this medication knowing that whether it will help is not certain and that you will need to help me assess its effectiveness. It will be helpful for you to read as much as you can about the medication and to monitor whether you see improvement in the symptoms that it's intended to affect. Will you do this?"

Provide Psychoeducation

See Video 1, Psychoeducation
See also section "Disclosure of the Diagnosis" in Chapter 3

Convey measured hope. Underscore that medications are adjunctive. Be open about the serious limitations of our knowledge about pharmacotherapy for borderline personality disorder (BPD) (see Table 6–1).

Show Concerned Attention

Appreciate patients' subjective distress—do not minimize. Being available for inquiries between sessions is helpful.

Emphasize the Need for Patient's Collaboration

Collaboration with patients is necessary to identify the goals (targets) for medications, to assess benefits, and to recognize side effects. Encourage patients to read and learn about medications and to become active monitors of whether target symptoms are changing (see Video 8, Managing Safety and Medications). This encourages thinking and a sense of agency.

Don't Ignore Negative Attitudes

Address the patient's negative attitudes 1) toward the prescribing physician (e.g., "You see me as a diagnosis, not as a person," "You ignore what I'm saying")

TABLE 6–1. **Current status of pharmacotherapy for borderline personality disorder (BPD)**

- About 30 randomized controlled trials have been conducted (antipsychotics > antidepressants > mood stabilizers > others), usually with small samples (average size about 40), variable outcome measures, and limited duration.

- No medication is uniformly or dramatically helpful.

- No drug has been licensed by the FDA as an effective treatment for BPD.

- Pharmaceutical company–sponsored research has been limited by disproportionate fears of violent or suicidal acts in patients who receive or do not receive medications—both incurring possible liability.

- Polypharmacy is associated with multiple side effects, and the effects of augmentation are unknown.

- The number of medications taken is inversely related to improvement.

- Minimal attention has been given to medication effects on interpersonal relationships.

---

or 2) about the hazards of medications (e.g., "I will lose myself," "I'll become a zombie"). Respond with both curiosity and reassurance.

Selecting Medications

Figure 6–1 is an algorithm for selecting medications; selection depends on the patient's motivation, symptom severity and type, and current medications. Be prepared to discuss the relative merits of different classes and types of medications (see Table 6–2), but note that medications might be helpful in decreasing anger and aggression but will usually have limited effects on depression or self-harm.

- **SSRIs**—uncertain or weak benefits, but safe with few side effects. Primarily useful for bona fide co-occurring major depressive disorder.
- **Tricyclic antidepressants (TCAs)**—uncertain or weak benefits, moderate side effects, and slow acting. Use normal doses, but be cautious in view of their potential lethality.
- **Mood stabilizers**—can help depressed mood, anger, and impulsivity but have limited effect on unstable affect. The patient should understand that psychotherapy is more helpful for affective instability. Mood stabilizers (lithium and valproate) may negatively affect libido and fetal health if the patient is pregnant. Topiramate and lamotrigine are safer than lithium. Use normal (bipolar disorder) doses.

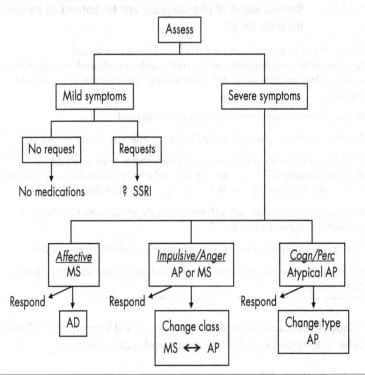

FIGURE 6–1.   Algorithm for medication choice for borderline personality disorder.

AD=antidepressant; AP=antipsychotic; MS=mood stabilizer; SSRI=selective serotonin reuptake inhibitor.

Assess the following:
1. Patient's motivation
2. Symptom severity and type: anxiety/depression/affective instability, impulsive/anger, cognitive/perceptual (Cogn/Perc)
3. Current medications

If patient is severely distressed or insistent, proceed as follows:
1. Affectively unstable, anxious/depressed—start with MS (e.g., topiramate or lamotrigine), move to AD (e.g., SSRIs)
2. Impulsive/anger—start with APs (e.g., aripiprazole or ziprasidone) or MS, move to the other class of medication
3. Cognitive/perceptual—start with APs, move to other types

- **Antipsychotics**—good for anger and impulse control but can be sedating and require self-discipline to avoid weight gain. Typical and atypical antipsychotics have similar effects. Of the atypical antipsychotics, aripiprazole and ziprasidone cause less weight gain than do olanzapine and quetiapine. Start with low doses and gradually increase. Encourage tapering and discontinuance after stability is achieved (often 2–4 weeks).

TABLE 6–2. Symptom targets and medication types

	Mood instability	Depression	Anxiety	Anger	Impulsivity	Cognitive/ perceptual
Selective serotonin reuptake inhibitors	?	+	?	?	+	–
Tricyclic antidepressants	–	–	–	+	?	–
Mood stabilizers	+	?/+	?	++	++	–
Antipsychotics	+	?	+	+	+	++
Anxiolytics	?	–	?	–	–	?

Note. ++=helpful; +=modestly helpful; ?=uncertain; –=negative.

Source. Adapted from Mercer et al. 2009; Silk and Faurino 2012.

- **Anxiolytics**—can decrease anxiety, but these medications can sedate, prompt behavioral outbursts that can negatively affect work and relationships, and evoke dependency (i.e., BPD patients have great difficulty with withdrawal after chronic use). Their use should be only intermittent to manage crises.

Comorbidities

See Video 3, Establishing an Alliance

BPD usually co-occurs with several other psychiatric disorders (see Table 6–3). Because modern psychiatrists are generally comfortable and capable within their role as psychopharmacologists and less comfortable and well trained in conducting psychosocial interventions, BPD psychopathology is often given secondary or no attention. This handbook addresses the training issue: every professional who assumes responsibility for a borderline patient should have acquired basic competence—should be comfortable and capable—in their role as treater; that is, "good enough." Part of basic competence is to know when BPD should take priority.

Selecting the Primary Diagnostic Target

As soon as the borderline diagnosis is made, clinicians need to be thoughtful about which of their patient's several disorders should become the primary target. Table 6–3 sets forth guidelines based on what remains an admittedly weak body of scientific evidence (J.G. Gunderson, R.L. Stout, M.T. Shea, et al., "Interactions of Borderline Personality Disorder and Mood Disorders Over Ten Years," unpublished manuscript, November 2013; Keuroghlian et al. 2013). Some summary conclusions follow:

- Treat BPD's comorbid disorders as primary targets when their presence precludes involvement or active learning (social and cognitive) (e.g., substance abuse, mania, complex posttraumatic stress disorder) or when motivation is lacking (antisocial personality disorder, anorexia). It is notable that of these disorders, only mania involves a primarily medicinal intervention.
- Treat BPD as the primary treatment target when the co-occurring disorder is unlikely to remit or is likely to relapse unless BPD is in remission (major depressive disorder, panic disorder, remitted bipolar I or bipolar II disorder, bulimia). It bears reiterating that making BPD the primary target does not preclude trials with medications appropriate for the co-occurring disorder (see Case 1, Roger, in Chapter 8 ["Case Illustrations"]).

For more discussion of comorbidity, see Chapter 3.

TABLE 6–3. Borderline personality disorder (BPD) comorbidity: which disorder is primary?

Disorder	% in BPD	% BPD in other disorders	BPD primary?	Reason
Major depressive disorder	50	15	Yes	Will remit if BPD does
Bipolar disorder	15	15		
Manic			No	Unable to use BPD treatment
Not manic			Yes	Recurrence ↓ if BPD remits
Bipolar II			Yes	Will remit if BPD does
Panic disorder	50	7	Yes	Will remit if BPD does
Posttraumatic stress disorder	30	8		
Early onset (complex)			No	Too vigilant to attach/be challenged
Adult onset			?	Able to use BPD treatment?
Substance use disorder	35	10	No	3–6 months of sobriety make BPD treatment feasible
Antisocial personality disorder	25	25	?	Is treatment for secondary gain?
Narcissistic personality disorder	15	25	Yes	↓BPD response to treatment but improves if BPD does
Eating disorder	20	20		
Anorexia			No	Unable to use BPD treatment
Bulimia			?	Is physical health stable?

Common Problems

Your Patient Resists Discontinuing Medications Despite Their Uncertain or Absent Benefits

Borderline patients and treaters often judge medicines differently (see Cowdry and Gardner 1988). Be firm and consistent in your judgment, but bow to patients' insistence on continuation unless, of course, side effects are dangerous. Also, cite as your policy that you routinely decrease and taper medications with uncertain benefits and restore them if they prove to have been effective.

Use of Medications for an Acutely Agitated or Potentially Self-Harming Patient

Treaters are particularly reluctant to administer medications to patients with acute agitation and potential suicidality because of concern about overdose or noncompliance. Although no empirical support exists for medication effectiveness in decreasing deliberate self-harm or suicidality, there may be "transferential" benefits in prescribing. Within acute situations, the short-term benefits from medications have not been and are unlikely to be measured.

Before prescribing, whenever possible, first involve the patient's other treaters and the patient's partner or family to explore alternative interventions and to gain their support. Then, if you have a good alliance and the patient offers reassurance that you can trust, consider giving your patient a limited (1-day) prescription for sedation (e.g., chlorpromazine, quetiapine, or olanzapine), and ask the patient to call you. Even if successful, this option should be identified as an exception, and after the crisis, an alternative plan should be established for any such future crises.

Your Patient Refuses Medications

Start by reassuring the patient that he or she can get better, even dramatically, without medications. Note, however, that medications, if used judiciously, might help and that if the patient improves, the value of medications will, unlike with most other psychiatric disorders, diminish (become obsolete). Do not expect the patient to agree with you immediately, or if, at your urging, he or she does agree to take medications, accept that he or she will remain wary. "Non-pushy," nonauthoritarian messages are apt to bring about an attitude change.

Your Patient Wants to Be Treated Only for a Chief Complaint of Depression

See Video 3, Establishing an Alliance
See also Case 3, April, in Chapter 8

The co-occurrence of major depressive disorder symptoms and BPD is usual (about 50%, 80% lifetime, with nearly 100% having chronic dysphoria). Understandably, treating the depression is often a patient's highest priority. However, even if you agree to introduce medications (probably a mood stabilizer; see Figure 6–1), the patient should be informed that BPD's improvement is more strongly associated with improvement in major depressive disorder than vice versa (Gunderson et al. 2004, submitted). Medications cannot fulfill the patient's need to "get a life." Those with genuine and severe co-occurring major depressive disorder are more apt to respond than are those whose depression is less severe and whose symptoms are weighted toward shame, loneliness, emptiness, or badness. Thus, you establish reasonable expectations and the importance of pursuing psychosocial therapies because effectiveness is more likely and more enduring.

Your Patient Has Received a Bipolar Disorder Diagnosis and Treatment With Mood Stabilizers

Patients with a bipolar diagnosis who are then identified as having BPD usually have persisting impulsivity and emotionality (usually inappropriate and excessive anger) that have not responded to prior treatment with mood stabilizers. You do not need to disagree with the bipolar diagnosis, but as per Figure 6–1, patients probably should try a different (nonbenzodiazepine) class (i.e., antipsychotic) of medications.

CHAPTER 7
Split Treatments

Rationale

Patients with borderline personality disorder (BPD) often have handicaps that exceed any one clinician's time and abilities (e.g., needs help finding a suitable school or work, has a family too disruptive or too dependent, has an inadequate safety net, insists on a trial of evidence-based treatment). Combining your therapeutic skills with those of another treater or modality is usually helpful when possible and when the resulting treatment is structured correctly (see Table 7–1). When done well, split treatments decrease burden, acting-out of anger (from self-harming behaviors to lateness), dropping out, and noncompliance.

Selecting Another Modality

Split treatments should give patients the benefits of two modalities (see Table 7–2); combining two individual therapists, for example, is rarely wise. The most common form of split treatment is a psychiatrist (or sometimes a primary care physician) who administers medications combined with an individual psychotherapist. This arrangement is fundamentally sound with two cautions: 1) it can easily fail when the physician ("too busy") fails to stay in touch with the therapist, and 2) psychiatrists should not reflexively assume referral to a psychotherapist is needed.

Within the Good Psychiatric Management (GPM) model, psychiatrists usually assume both of these roles, consult a psychopharmacologist when necessary, and add another modality as a second treatment. The choice of a second modality should be carefully considered. For psychiatrists who see their borderline patients every few weeks or less, or for psychotherapists who are psychodynamically dedicated (and disinclined or inexperienced

TABLE 7–1.	Framework for split treatments for borderline patients

- One treater is "primary"—manages safety, evaluates progress, authorizes treatment changes

- Treaters will communicate at their discretion—always about safety, noncompliance

- Treaters need to understand and respect each other's complementary roles

with case management), the best partner in split treatment is someone who does case management. This role involves being advisory and supportive and can include community interventions (e.g., locating apartments, overseeing budget, use of public transportation, conjoint meetings with roommates). The most available and least expensive other modality is a self-help organization such as Alcoholics Anonymous, Narcotics Anonymous, or Eating Disorders Anonymous. Still, when available, the most complementary second modality is group therapy (see section "Group Therapy" later in this chapter).

Common Problems

Your Patient Devalues the Other Treater (As Useless or Cruel)

A basic rule of split treatments is neither to validate nor to object to complaints about the other treater. This does not mean being neutral; express concern and explore what led to the hostile and dismissive reaction. Usually, one knows the co-treater, and if the complaint is clearly paranoid or easily correctable, a co-treater should state that it seems implausible or that the allegation seems unlikely on the basis of experience (see Case 6, Melanie, in Chapter 8 ["Case Illustrations"]). In any event, it is in any borderline patient's interest to make a complaint directly to the offending treater. This offers an opportunity for an important corrective experience: it is an exercise in self-assertion (and self-agency) and should correct their preconceptions insofar as the other treater fails to react by withdrawing or becoming angry. If the patient refuses to talk to the other treater, arrange for a conjoint meeting with the other treater and the patient. When a patient refuses even this option, it is often best to make this nonnegotiable. This is most clearly indicated when the patient is potentially dangerous to himself or herself, when the other treater is the primary therapist (or the other treatment is otherwise deemed essential, e.g., Alcoholics Anonymous [AA] or family therapy), or when the remaining treater feels burdened by too much responsibility. When you are the primary treater and the patient will not address any com-

TABLE 7–2. **Complementary functions of different modalities**

Modality	Functions
Individual psychotherapy	Clarifying and validating a sense of self; learning to think first and to recognize cause-and-effect patterns; also offers corrective experiences (see section "How Change Occurs" in Chapter 2)
Case management	Activities of daily living, work and family initiatives, budget, diet, etc.
Medication management	Can address subjective distress; medical training helps with co-occurring medical issues; can facilitate hospitalization (see Chapter 6 ["Pharmacotherapy and Comorbidity"])
Group therapy	Social skills, self-awareness, self-disclosure, empathy, affect tolerance (see section "Group Therapy" in this chapter)
Family interventions (usually not patients and parents together)	Decrease situational stress, increase support (see section "Family Interventions" in this chapter)
Self-help groups	Social (support), self-disclosure

plaints to the other treater, you might insist on adding another treater. Accepting a patient's refusal to address the complaints to the other therapist is never helpful!

The Physician Who Prescribes Medications Does Not Respond to Your Communications

When the prescribing physician often does not respond to communications, the psychotherapist (or other psychosocial therapist) usually becomes reconciled, knowing that the psychiatrist or physician often has competing responsibilities. Although this arrangement is not ideal, it can work if the noncommunicative physician 1) defers to you, 2) retains a narrow role, and 3) uses relevant information from you (e.g., patient complains of insomnia, weakness, or anxiety). The physician who disregards your feedback or uses his or her authority to opine about other parts of the patient's care needs to be reminded that he or she should first discuss such issues with you. If physicians do not do this, and their interventions are harmful, they need to be advised to stop before you recommend that your patient work with someone else. Should that fail, advise both your patient and the offending physician that you are unable to continue under the circumstances.

Your Co-Treater Is Not Adhering to the Frame

You learn, for example, that your co-treater has failed to inform you of your patient's intent to dismiss you, or has encouraged the patient to stop attending groups, or is taking an extended leave. You need to discuss this failure and, if it persists, ask for consultation. If the primary treater tells the negligent treater to terminate, he or she often angrily resists, and the patient then must choose. It is harmful to patients to have a protracted dysfunctional or hostile partnership.

Group Therapy (Including Dialectical Behavior Therapy Skills Groups)

See Case 5, Lawrence, in Chapter 8

Groups are underused. Because most borderline patients do not want to do group therapy, clinicians need to actively promote their use.

> "Group therapies offer lessons that can't be learned from individual psychotherapy. Specifically, groups demonstrate that others have similar problems and have different ways of coping with them. Group therapies will also highlight how you impede making the close relationships that you want, and they can help you change those patterns. Moreover, in group therapies you can learn to listen when people express feelings you usually avoid and you can learn to understand why people have those feelings. I consider this the single most cost-beneficial therapy available."

Most borderline patients instinctively resist participation. They fear what others will think or say about them, and some do not want to share attention. If the primary therapist openly endorses a group therapy and actively communicates with the group therapist, this resistance diminishes and can usually resolve. For many treaters in office practice, group therapies may not seem to be easily available. Calling local mental health clinics for access to their groups may be all that is required. Virtually any group that is structured and has an active leader will be helpful. Table 7–3 offers a guide to types of group therapy.

Most widely available are AA or other self-help groups that can serve many of the same functions as professionally led groups. Because group therapies are so useful and cost-effective for borderline patients, participation should be required in outpatient clinic settings.

For some borderline patients, individual therapy is nonproductive unless the problems in social living are being forced into their attention by group

TABLE 7–3. Hierarchy[a] of group therapies for borderline patients

Type of group	Emphases
Self-help	Support, social networking, clarity, simplicity
Self-assessment	Support, self-disclosure, listening, activities of daily living
Skills building (Dialectical Behavior Therapy skills are the preeminent exemption)	Didactic, self-regulatory skills primary with secondary social skills building
Interpersonal	Closeness, trust

[a]In terms of availability, costs, and capability of patients.

(or family) sessions. If such patients refuse to enter or attend groups, it may be necessary to make individual psychotherapy contingent on this. Because borderline patients' offending interpersonal behaviors are often more evident—and more readily challenged—within group therapies, the primary therapist needs to be aware and actively integrate those problems into the individual psychotherapy.

Skills Training Groups

Group therapies that see borderline patients' interpersonal and functional problems as social learning handicaps adopt a training-like approach to correcting these. Within this approach, Dialectical Behavior Therapy (DBT) skills training groups are by far the most widely available and empirically validated. Skills training groups teach patients more adaptive ways of coping with problems such as misattributions, impulsivity, intolerance of aloneness, or excessive anger. Such groups are structured, require active and directive leadership, and are generally less stressful for borderline patients than are other types of groups. There is no inherent incompatibility between skills training groups and other forms of treatment. Problems can arise, however, when the purveyor of the other (usually individual) therapy fails to understand and respect the value of skills training. This basic failure dooms any split treatment but perhaps attained more notoriety from an earlier generation of psychoanalysts who were critical of the concepts of social handicaps and hostile to DBT. The only inherent tension for GPM with DBT skills groups is the relatively greater emphasis DBT (or other skills training groups) gives to controlling emotions via distraction compared with GPM's greater emphasis on increasing awareness and tolerance of emotions.

Common Problems (Groups)

Hostile, Dismissive, or Nonparticipatory Behaviors Within Sessions

Some patients will not listen to others, dominate, or are rude. After interrupting and identifying the objectionable behaviors, the group leader invites others' responses. (Group leaders *must* be active; see subsection "Be Active, Not Reactive" in "Basic Therapeutic Approach" section of Chapter 2 ["Overall Principles"].) If their feedback also does not change the disruptive behaviors, the leader will need to disinvite the member, stating that he or she "just isn't ready."

Exclusionary Alliances Between Group Members

Alliances usually occur when group members meet outside of groups. Social involvement between group members outside sessions is often helpful, but when it involves a sexual relationship, includes drug use, or is otherwise exclusionary, as a matter of policy, the group leader needs to openly discuss this within the context of the group. This can be prompted by other patients' complaints or by the exclusionary behaviors within the group (e.g., two members sit side by side and either do not participate or carry on private comments to each other). Intersession relationships that interfere with participation in the group also should be addressed within subsequent group sessions and may require one or both being suspended. Educational comments about how the wish for exclusive and exclusionary relationships is a symptom of borderline personality disorder that accounts for their problems sustaining relationships may get everyone involved in challenging the behaviors without scapegoating those who are enacting this.

Absences

With the exception of absences due to hospitalization or illness, repeated absences that are willful should be discussed within the group, and if this fails to improve attendance, the leader, after discussion with the primary treater, should suspend the patient with an invitation to reapply if she or he feels more committed.

Family Interventions

See Video 9, Managing Family Involvement

"You have a handicapped child. We know that the problems we encounter in treating your child are those that you have struggled with for a long time. By learning new ways of responding to your child's handicaps, with what we call 'counterintuitive parenting' you can improve communications, diminish alienation, and improve your child's progress."

An intake session with the patient accompanied by parents usually identifies serious conflicts. Getting the parents involved as collaborators begins here (for an illustration, see Case 7, Jill, in Chapter 8). Table 7–4 describes the types of family interventions and the indications for their use. All parents or spouses should receive basic psychoeducation (see Table 3–2 in Chapter 3 ["Making the Diagnosis"]). This usually opens the door for counseling about improved parenting skills or support groups. Family therapy can be valuable, but families first need to be able to listen and to identify a systems problem they all wish to work on. Such families are unfortunately the exception rather than the rule.

Enlisting Patient Support for Parent or Spouse Participation

Borderline patients often oppose family involvement until they are told that its objectives are to help their parents to understand them better and become more supportive and less stress inducing. These are quite desirable goals from the patient's borderline perspective.

Enlisting Parental Participation

Supportive participation by parents (or spouses) is often essential for creating an adequate "holding" environment (see Chapter 2). Most parents feel helpless and frustrated. Many are suspicious or skeptical about treatment. These attitudes usually can be reversed with education and empathy. Treaters should acknowledge that the parents' problems with their child are the same as those faced within treatments and that these problems are the targets for change in the treatment being offered. Parents always know that what they have been doing has not worked. Your help offers welcome relief to their burden.

Alliance Building

Three forms of alliance-building interventions—support, psychoeducation, and inviting collaboration—are all easily provided and rarely fail (see also section "Building an Alliance" in Chapter 4 ["Getting Started"]).

• *Support*—family members experience chronic stress, emotional distress, and financial burden. Learn about their concerns; listen to their fears of suicide and their feelings of hopelessness. Acknowledge that you know that they have done the best they could. Tell parents that their offspring

TABLE 7–4.   Hierarchy[a] of family interventions for borderline patients

Type of intervention	Features	Comments
Psychoeducation	Initial focus is about the disorder (see Table 3–2 in Chapter 3) and should be offered to all parents and spouses. Subsequent focus is about parenting.	For basic family guidelines, see Appendix D.
Counseling	Review family guidelines, advise, and problem solve.	Families usually welcome these sessions.
Support groups	Multiple family groups, "Family Connections"[b]	Helpful if available; clinics should develop.
Conjoint sessions (patient and parents)	Can be led by family counselor, primary clinician, or both. Useful for planning and problem-solving issues such as budget, sleep hygiene, treatment adherence, emergencies, vacations.	Can be very helpful in sustaining the holding environment and to decrease splitting.
Family therapy	Reserved for patients and parents who can discuss conflicts without interrupting, having angry outbursts, or leaving.	Parent blaming can be useful only if parents can accept with regrets whatever is true in the borderline patient's allegations.

[a]In terms of availability, breadth of identity, and costs.
[b]Sponsored by National Education Alliance for Borderline Personality Disorder/National Alliance on Mental Illness.

with BPD should be seen as a "special needs" child who will not respond well to usual parenting; what was good for them or for their other children can unwittingly be harmful to their offspring with BPD.

• *Psychoeducation (see also Video 1)*—This begins with the disorder (see Table 3–2), then encourage reading the "Guidelines for Families" (see Appendix D) or other educational materials. Offering a description of the interaction of genes and environmental adversity helps counter reductionist ideas about a diseased child or a destructive family. The following illustrates how explaining this interaction can be done:

"Like other major psychiatric illnesses, the origin of borderline personality disorder is significantly heritable: it is safe to say it is more than 50%. This places it above depression and anxiety disorders, but less than schizophrenia. This means that to develop BPD requires a significant genetic disposition. It also means that it would be difficult to develop the disorder without significant environmental adversity. What the pre-BPD child has inherited isn't clear. The two major candidates are either excessive emotionality or [as described here]), excessive interpersonal reactivity [see Chapter 2, first section, and Chapter 3, section "How to Disclose"]. Such a disposition makes this a difficult child to parent.

"When a child develops BPD, parents always wonder whether they are to blame. The fact that genetics are involved can diminish that concern, but it doesn't really dismiss the contribution of parental behaviors and of family environment more generally.

"Easily stressed or anxious parents will find it difficult to parent a pre-borderline child. Being reactive or emotional might be inconsequential with a more easy-to-please child, but these qualities will doubtless aggravate the pre-BPD infant. The point here is that children greatly influence parenting—as much as vice versa. It might take an extremely calm and involved parent to quell the otherwise disturbing emotional expressions and sensitivity to separations or anger that characterize a pre-borderline infant.

"The causal effect of childhood trauma is often a concern. About 65% of borderline patients report neglect and either physical or sexual abuse. Such experiences no doubt contribute to BPD's etiology, but they are neither necessary nor sufficient. Many children exposed to such experiences grow up without psychiatric sequelae. The pre-borderline person will have more severe reactions, feel less able to discuss his or her experience, and have more enduring consequences due to inherited disposition."

• *Collaboration*—encourage parents to become an actively collaborating part of the treatment effort. They should provide basic support for treatment. Their complaints or questions or those of their BPD family member about treatment should be addressed directly to the treaters. They should provide basic support for the patient: the child is handicapped by interpersonal hypersensitivity and limited self-control. They also should not take their borderline child's anger or blame too personally. This is hard, but they should try not to fight back when criticized.

Common Problems (Family)

Your Patient Refuses to Allow Contact With Parents or Spouse

Even if your patient is an adult without financial dependence and without an apparent risk of suicide (or homicide), parents and spouses still should be encouraged to advise treaters of their concerns and to know about their credentials and perception of progress. If your patient is an adolescent or is an adult with financial dependence on his or her parents, assure the patient of confidentiality, then firmly but gently state that attaining his or her parents' perspectives and support is necessary. (See subsections "Patient Refuses to Accept the Framework" in Chapter 4 and "Your Patient With Dangerous Suicidal or Self-Harming Behaviors Refuses to Give You Permission to Contact Significant Others" in Chapter 5 ["Managing Suicidality and Nonsuicidal Self-Harm"].)

Patient Alleges Sexual or Physical Abuse (Within Family)

Meetings with the accused parent should be sought. Patients who object may either be fearful (rightly occasionally but usually unrealistically) or be making false allegations. The issue is often best addressed by meeting with other family members. Parents who are guilty often will not want to participate in conjoint meetings with their offspring. Sometimes even guilty parents will support treatments if they believe that their offspring will not disclose this history or are in high denial themselves. Clinicians should be sympathetic to such allegations but should be careful not to validate either their occurrence or the parent's toxicity. Vilification of innocent parents or encouraging the patient's identity as a victim can both tragically perpetuate alienation and contribute to chronicity.

Families Are Held Hostage by Fears of Suicide or Other Self-Harm

Fear that the patient may commit suicide or other self-harm can be sustained and progressive. The "specialness" of both the problem child and the parents' self-image as heroic caregivers complicates efforts to change these situations. Parents should be advised that assuming such responsibility is harmful to their offspring and to themselves and other family members. Moving out of this situation is facilitated by relocating the BPD offspring to a hospital or a residential setting, including sometimes even a responsible—and willing!—relative. This gives time for the offspring to get involved in treatment and for the parents to learn new ways of managing suicidal threats on their offspring's return. When such options are not available, the transition needs to be done gradually with the therapist as an intermediary—often requiring multiple conjoint sessions. Suicidal gestures are likely to occur, which will test the families' resolve—and their capability—not to overreact and to respond with moderation.

Parents are Uninterested or Disrespectful

Once you have told parents what to do (e.g., listen, seek support) and what not to do (e.g., escalate fights, ignore suicidal ideation, "manage" crises without informing you), and the parents disregard your admonitions, then you can validate the patient's complaints about these parental failures (i.e., parental abrogation of their reasonably expectable responsibilities). Becoming reconciled to such dysfunctional parenting then becomes the challenge.

Parents Are Estranged From Each Other

Gaining supportive involvement from parents who are estranged from each other may be difficult and time-consuming. Each parent may need your attention and education delivered separately. When they sacrifice or neglect what's best for their BPD child because of their anger toward each other, this should be made explicit. If it continues, then (as in the previous discussion of disinterested or disrespectful parents) helping the child become reconciled to this problem becomes the therapeutic challenge.

SECTION III

GPM Workbook

Case Illustrations

CHAPTER 8
Case Illustrations

Each of the following case illustrations will highlight the application of the Good Psychiatric Management (GPM) treatment model as well as common problems that clinicians confront. The case vignettes are interrupted by **Decision Points.** Upon reaching such points, readers are encouraged to consider how they might respond to the clinical situation. A section follows the case vignette in which possible **Alternative Responses** to the Decision Points are identified. There are, of course, many other responses that might occur and might be helpful. The reader is asked to consider whether the given response is good, i.e., *will be helpful* (scored as **1**). If the reader concludes the response is *possibly helpful but with persistent reservations* (because it depends on other considerations or because the response's effect seems unpredictable), then the rating is **2**. For those responses that a reader considers *not helpful—or even harmful,* the rating should be **3**.

After completing the ratings, the reader will find the merits of the proposed alternative responses considered in a section called **Discussion.** Here reference is made to sections of the manual that are pertinent, although in many instances the manual has not covered all of the specific problems identified in these cases. Still, the Handbook's general principles should offer useful guides.

Case 1, Roger: Trouble in College

Illustrating Chapter 3 ("Making the Diagnosis"), Chapter 4 ("Getting Started"), and Chapter 6 ("Pharmacotherapy and Comorbidity")

It is difficult to disentangle the contributions of borderline personality disorder (BPD) from those of other psychiatric conditions and developmental crises, but it is certainly clear that in this case, a socially naive young man becomes self-destructive and dysfunctional when he leaves home for college and his first romance.

Case Vignette

Roger, a 21-year-old man, comes to see you with his parents for a diagnostic consultation and treatment recommendations after two unsuccessful attempts at college and a referral from his primary care physician.

Roger is a Peruvian-born only child adopted 4 weeks after birth and raised in rural Pennsylvania by an artist mother and a father who is a computer programmer. As a child, he was sensitive and "clingy." His psychiatric history is significant for long-standing attention-deficit/hyperactivity disorder (ADHD) symptoms, and his parents report that he did well while taking stimulants (primarily Adderall) until he left for college. He is quite bright and earned nearly all A's in high school and completed some 40 college credits while there. His life in high school was consumed primarily by studies (he read voraciously), the school jazz band, and a few intense friendships. In retrospect, he tells you that he always felt very insecure and believed that he was "different."

When he left home to attend college, things began to deteriorate. He met a group of friends who emphasized respect for the environment and stressed living a "natural" life; he stopped using stimulants (Adderall) after he adopted their critical stance toward medication. He struggled academically for the first time, and his parents became concerned by his severe self-criticism. He had a first girlfriend. He reported that he thought she was "perfect, my everything, an angel," and she made him feel there was hope for him "to actually feel like I'm likeable." He spent much of his time with her or thinking about her. Roger cut himself for the first time when she threatened to end the relationship "because I was too jealous." He subsequently cut himself four more times, always when he felt threatened by her suggestions that the relationship was "imperfect" or "not necessarily permanent." He told you, "If she had felt toward me like I felt about her, I wouldn't need to be here talking to you." The first time they broke up was the week before finals in his freshman year, and he drank in his dorm room for 9 consecutive days, failing all of his finals and two of his four classes.

That summer, Roger returned home and took up residence in his basement, where he stayed up all night reading and smoking cigarettes. When he refused to return to school, his parents took him to his primary care physician, who diagnosed depression and started citalopram (20 mg) for depression. He has continued taking it without obvious benefit, but he said that he likes "taking something to help my mind." He eventually did return to college, where he fruitlessly pursued his former girlfriend, cut himself three more times, and barely made it through the semester.

In your initial interview, Roger presented as a tall, pale young man with long hair who seemed somewhat suspicious and distracted. You found him a bit tough to follow—he was circumstantial and unfocused. This was surprising given his past academic success. He was most concerned by his ongoing struggles with depression, characterized by little interest in school or activities, persistent guilty ruminations, difficulty with sleep initiation, and recurrent passive thoughts of dying by slitting his wrists in the bath. He has never acted on those thoughts (and does not intend to). On questioning, he noted a period of sleeplessness and high energy during finals of his first semester of college, where he was awake for 88 hours (his friends counted it up and were concerned). He also remembered that during this period, he wrote all of his papers "very well" and played his saxophone the "best ever." You consider the complications of this diagnostic picture. [**Decision Point 1**]

With the benefit of further questions and collateral information, you conclude that Roger has three disorders: ADHD, bipolar II disorder, and BPD. After reviewing the criteria together, Roger and his family endorse all three diagnoses. You are unclear how much of Roger's decline in function is due to discontinuation of stimulant treatment for ADHD and how much is related to the BPD stressors of separation and rejection. With these issues in mind, you formulate an approach to Roger's treatment. [**Decision Point 2**]

To frame Roger and his family's expectations for treatment, you provide psychoeducation about BPD. [**Decision Point 3**] You describe how your treatment approach for ADHD and bipolar II will be influenced by BPD comorbidity. [**Decision Point 4**] Roger resisted your effort to involve him in making decisions, but after discussion, you both decided to stop citalopram and to start atomoxetine (Strattera).

A week later, Roger and his parents describe considerable improvement. He has cleaned and shortened his hair, and he is much more organized and linear in his thinking. He wants to see you weekly. In the next few weeks, he called his ex-girlfriend to tell her that he will not be contacting her any more, and he "de-friended" some 476 Facebook friends who reminded him of "bad" parts of his life. He tells you that you're the best doctor he has found, and he is now very hopeful that he can get back on track—return to college. This is good news, and you consider how to respond to his improvement. [**Decision Point 5**]

Decision Points: Alternative Responses

(1 = will be helpful, 2 = possibly helpful, continuing reservations, 3 = not helpful—or even harmful)
See next subsection for discussion.

1. Diagnostically, your initial thinking on Roger is that

    A. BPD explains Roger's presenting issues, and it warrants disclosure of the diagnosis to the patient. ___

B. The patient likely has ADHD, and this should be further assessed and treated. ___

C. Roger's depression combined with 88 hours of wakefulness establishes a bipolar disorder. ___

2. Having established the BPD, ADHD, and bipolar II diagnoses, you conclude that

A. In the absence of training on treatment of BPD, you should confine your role to treating the other two diagnoses. ___

B. BPD's treatment should be the first priority. ___

C. Hopes for a good medication response should be qualified. ___

D. You should enlist Roger in evaluating effects of his drug therapies. ___

3. Psychoeducation about BPD should include

A. BPD is a genetically based "brain disease." ___

B. Treatment of BPD is optional because its natural course is to get better. ___

C. Encouragement of strategies to reduce exposure to interpersonal stress. ___

4. Comorbidity with BPD affects your treatment approach for ADHD and bipolar II disorder as follows:

A. Because the patient has BPD (and bipolar II), great care should be exercised in prescribing a stimulant. ___

B. It is reasonable to continue citalopram. ___

C. You should start lithium to stabilize the patient's mood. ___

D. You should assess the status of Roger's relationship with you and his attitude about the proposed medication changes. ___

5. Response to Roger's improvement and enthusiasm about you should include the following:

A. Advise him to find a therapist experienced with BPD and confine yourself to managing his medications. ___

B. Provide basic education about BPD and psychotherapy and discuss how he would like you to help him. ___

C. Agree to work with the patient weekly, and refer Roger and his family for family therapy with a colleague you know well who specializes in adoption issues. ___

Discussion

1. Diagnostically, your initial thinking on Roger is that

   (see "Disclosure of the Diagnosis" in Chapter 3; see also Chapter 6)

   A. BPD explains Roger's presenting issues and warrants disclosure of the diagnosis to the patient. [3] (The patient's presentation warrants consideration of other diagnoses, i.e., ADHD and bipolar disorder. Moreover, the BPD diagnosis requires more exploration of the criteria before it can be confidently established. His problems with rejection sensitivity, exclusive attachment, and self-injury after interpersonal stress strongly suggest BPD. However, you should ask more about other criteria such as anger, splits [black-or-white, all-or-nothing], interpersonal splits [he idealizes; does he devalue?], and emptiness.)
   B. The patient likely has ADHD, and this should be further assessed and treated. [1] (Yes, the history and presentation are suggestive. In addition, you need to review past neuropsychological test results. Initiating a successful treatment of Roger's ADHD can be alliance-building and might help increase cortical controls for BPD's interpersonal sensitivity.)
   C. Roger's depression combined with 88 hours of wakefulness establishes a bipolar disorder. [2] (It seems probable, but first you must determine whether the period of wakefulness was substance induced and whether bipolarity is confirmed by other periods of energy enhancement, elation, and increased productivity.)

2. Having established the BPD, ADHD, and bipolar II diagnoses, you conclude that

   (see Chapter 2 ["Overall Principles"], Chapter 4, and Chapter 6)

   A. In the absence of training on treatment of BPD, you should confine your role to treating the other two diagnoses. [3] (No. As this handbook notes, basic knowledge about BPD, common sense, and an attentive encouraging attitude are sufficient to help most borderline patients very significantly.)
   B. BPD's treatment should be the first priority. [3] (In terms of management of the patient's mood, cutting, and interpersonal symptoms, the primary target is the BPD. Still, the degree to which Roger's decline is related to a discontinued stimulant is unclear,

and this should become the first priority. He is an intelligent young man who is unfocused and cannot function at college! Missing this piece would have negative effects on the patient's life, and stimulants might have dramatic and immediate benefits.)

C. Hopes for a good medication response should be qualified. [2] (This becomes important whenever a mood disorder co-occurs with BPD. "Overselling" the benefits of medications for mood would be a mistake.)

D. You should enlist Roger in evaluating effects of his drug therapies. [1] (Helping Roger learn to assess the effects of medication on his rejection sensitivity, mood, and attention is a way you can help the patient learn to attend to his inner life and become active in taking control of his life.)

3. Psychoeducation about BPD should include

(see "Disclosure of the Diagnosis" in Chapter 3)

A. BPD is a genetically based "brain disease." [2] (It is important for both patients and their families to know that this disorder has very significant genetic determinants. By itself, however, this message invites a passive fatalism that is harmful. It is important that they recognize that the adaptations Roger made to the genetic disposition are environmentally determined—and that Roger and his family can effect changes in those adaptations with time and effort.)

B. Treatment of BPD is optional because its natural course is to get better. [3] (The natural course of BPD does convey hope; it also conveys warnings. BPD has a range of outcomes; many people with BPD do not achieve good interpersonal or functional outcomes. Good treatment enhances both the likelihood and the speed of recovery. It would be shortsighted to not encourage Roger to use informed treatments—including Good Psychiatric Management [GPM].)

C. Encouragement of strategies to reduce exposure to interpersonal stress. [2] (When exposures are unnecessary [e.g., a highly critical boss, an abusive partner, a drunken parent], borderline patients should be encouraged to find more supportive social settings. Roger's stressor, an overstimulating romance, might be hard to avoid in the long term. In the short term, he would certainly benefit from psychoeducation—that is, underscoring how he should "practice" with dating and that seeking an exclusive romance is inherently unlikely to succeed. The goals of treatment are to help BPD patients learn to tolerate such stressors better and to accept limitations in themselves and in others.)

4. Comorbidity with BPD affects your treatment approach for ADHD and bipolar II disorder as follows:

   (see Chapter 2 and Chapter 6)

   A. Because the patient has BPD (and bipolar II), great care should be exercised in prescribing a stimulant. [2] (Although the BPD diagnosis in and of itself does not mean that the patient is likely to misuse stimulants, sending a supply of them with Roger, especially were he to return to a college campus, might be risky. Moreover, despite his past success with Adderall, the risk for a switch to mania with stimulants warrants discussion; atomoxetine is probably preferable. The discussion, rather than the actual decision, is where the action is: it reinforces the treatment principles of thinking through problems and the need for Roger to take an active role in evaluating effects and in controlling his life.)

   B. It is reasonable to continue citalopram. [2] (Despite having made the diagnosis of bipolar II disorder, and despite the fact that Roger liked "taking something for his mind," polypharmacy, especially with an antidepressant, is potentially problematic. Helping the patient talk about the meaning of the medication and his prior treatment relationship are wise first steps. As in the previous point, the discussion is where the action is.)

   C. You should start lithium to stabilize the patient's mood. [3] (In a depression-predominant bipolar disorder with a history of one hypomanic episode, lamotrigine may be appropriate for mood stabilization and offer benefits for anger, anxiety, and affective symptoms with BPD. Given its potential for toxicity and lethality in overdose, lithium is usually less preferable.)

   D. You should assess the status of Roger's relationship with you and his attitude about the proposed medication changes. [1] (With borderline patients, it is unwise to prescribe medications without consideration of alliance, likely compliance, family support, and so on.)

5. Response to Roger's improvement and enthusiasm about you should include the following:

   (see Chapter 2, "Building an Alliance" in Chapter 4, and Chapter 6)

A. Advise him to find a therapist experienced with BPD and confine yourself to managing his medications. [3] (There could be good reasons for a split treatment with this complicated psychophar-macology/comorbidity picture, but his apparent idealization of you would be a poor reason to add another treater. Most BPD pa-tients do well without seeing a specialist. Given Roger's intent to return to school, you are likely to have a valuable role in helping him manage that stress.)

B. Provide basic education about BPD and psychotherapy and dis-cuss how he would like you to help him. [1] (Yes, regardless of what you decide treatment-wise, you are involving him in making choices and inviting him to "think first." It may be a significant task for Roger to identify goals for psychological change. At this point, his need for ongoing psychotherapy is unclear. It seems likely that he has responded so well to the resumed treatment of his ADHD that his proposed return to school is realistic and on-going case management will be sufficient.)

C. Agree to work with the patient weekly, and refer Roger and his family for family therapy with a colleague you know well who spe-cializes in adoption issues. [3] (Agreeing to see the patient in on-going treatment may be appropriate [see B above], but the proposal for family therapy and the focus on adoption issues are premature and potentially alienating at this stage.)

Case 2, Loretta: Late-Night Calls

Illustrating Chapter 2, Chapter 4, Chapter 5 ("Managing Suicidality and Nonsuicidal Self-Harm"), and Chapter 6

This vignette concerns shifting a borderline patient's complaints of anxiety and depression into fears of being alone. The treater is skillfully responsive, but not overreactive, to late-night calls.

Case Vignette

Loretta, a 27-year-old white woman, entered an outpatient clinic with com-plaints of depression and panic. Although she met criteria for both major de-pressive disorder and panic disorder, it was evident that these symptoms were superimposed on recurrent crises related to her drug-abusing boy-friend, Carl, and to a history of cutting that began in early adolescence tied to her stormy relationship with her first boyfriend. When you suggested that her interpersonal crises with Carl will need to be addressed, she looked ap-prehensive and said that she just hoped you'd help her feel better. [**Decision**

Point 1] After reviewing the criteria for BPD, Loretta said, "it was like looking in a mirror." The patient agreed to weekly visits, began a trial of lamotrigine, and, per your usual practice, was given your telephone number for emergencies. Several days later, she called to ask you about side effects. She was quickly reassured and was thankful.

At her second appointment, she hesitantly confided that she has insomnia that sometimes leads to panic attacks during which she feels "unsafe." She noted that these episodes have become more frequent recently. [**Decision Point 2**] After you expressed concern about this and made inquiries, you learned that her boyfriend has been out late, and she becomes panicky and unable to sleep when he's away. Loretta inquires, "If I ever need to, would it be all right to call you?" [**Decision Point 3**]

During the next 3 weeks, Loretta reliably comes early to her appointments. She begins to disclose a very troubled childhood in which her depressed mother was unavailable and her overworked father drank too much. Her adolescence was marked by stormy, unstable sexual relationships, but her self-esteem was sustained by being on the school soccer team and her excellence as a player. During the telling, she is appropriately emotional and seems to have become more trustful toward you. You feel a growing connection and sympathy toward her.

In this context, Loretta calls you at 11:30 P.M., shortly after you've fallen asleep. She is sobbing and difficult to understand. She recovers enough to tell you that her boyfriend, Carl, has angrily left their apartment. After a few minutes, she seems almost cheerful as she says that she's sorry to bother you. [**Decision Point 4**] You ask her if she's feeling better. She says "yes" and then adds, "but don't worry, I'm not suicidal." You say, "I'm glad you feel better" and "The fact that you can feel better after talking to me is a subject to consider in our next session." Then you say "good night." You return to bed feeling glad to be turned to and trusted and to have been helpful. You also wonder with irritation whether she really needed to call so late.

A few hours later, you are awakened by another call. Loretta is sobbing again, this time saying that she knows that you are actually angry and fears you won't want to see her in treatment. She begins to sob again, saying, "I don't know whether I can go on like this." [**Decision Point 5**] When she tells you that she's referring to her relationship with her boyfriend, you tell her that's a good topic to discuss at the next session. After this call, you have trouble getting back to sleep and irritably wonder whether you had mismanaged the earlier call—including whether she had intuited your irritation.

In the next session, Loretta enters with downcast eyes and says that she's sorry to have bothered you. She then describes the recurring turmoil in her relationships with Carl. She details recent fights they've had. It emerges that Carl is generally "sweet" and protective toward her, but he can have a "short fuse" whenever she is critical of him. She moves on to describe previous episodes with this pattern. [**Decision Point 6**] Loretta describes getting panicky when she feels rejected, convinced that no one cares, and then becoming desperate about being alone. She said that she felt reassured when you answered the telephone. "I don't remember exactly what you said, but I know it helped me a lot." [**Decision Point 7**]

Decision Points: Alternative Responses

(1 = will be helpful, 2 = possibly helpful, continuing reservations, 3 = not helpful—or even harmful)
See next subsection for discussion.

1. In response to Loretta's wish to be treated for her depression and
   anxiety, you should

   A. Agree to prioritize these symptoms. ___
   B. Tell her that she has BPD and this explains her symptoms. ___
   C. Ask her to review the criteria for BPD, noting that it might explain
      her symptoms. ___

2. In response to Loretta's insomnia and panic attacks, you should

   A. Begin a suicide risk assessment. ___
   B. Inquire whether these symptoms are related to problems with her
      boyfriend. ___
   C. Express concern and invite her to contact you before her anxiety
      escalates. ___
   D. Ask whether there is any way you could help. ___
   E. Express concern about whether the session with you had wors-
      ened these symptoms. ___
   F. Review possible medication changes. ___

3. When Loretta asks whether she might call you if she needs to, you
   should

   A. Discourage her from calling you. ___
   B. Inquire how she hopes talking with you could be helpful. ___
   C. Encourage her to use the local crisis hotline. ___
   D. Ask her to describe circumstances where she might "need" to call
      you. ___
   E. Note that she cannot count on you always being available, and
      discuss other ways that she can manage crises. ___

4. In response to Loretta's highly distressed 11:30 call, you should

   A. Empathize with her distress. ___
   B. Ask what she and her boyfriend fought about. ___
   C. Encourage her to breathe deeply and count to 100 when she has
      such episodes of panic. ___

D. Apologetically tell her that you were asleep, and offer her an additional appointment in the morning. ____

5. When Loretta calls again several hours later saying "I don't know whether I can go on like this," you should

A. Tell her to develop a safety plan. ____
B. Ask what her concern with "going on" refers to. ____
C. Encourage her to seek help at an emergency department. ____
D. Ask whether you had failed to be helpful in the prior call. ____
E. Inquire whether she has tried to reach her boyfriend. ____
F. Reassure her that you are not angry and that you plan to work with her for as long as it takes. ____

6. In the next session, when Loretta describes her recurrent crises with Carl, you should

A. Listen carefully and encourage her to talk more about this issue. ____

B. Interrupt her discussion of the relationship and ask her to discuss what occurred during the telephone call. ____
C. Note how the hostile dependent relationship with Carl is similar to what she has described with her parents. ____
D. Ask her whether calling you had been helpful and, if so, why. ____
E. Indicate that having your sleep disrupted was irritating but that you were also glad to be helpful. ____
F. Consider other ways to deal with this should the situation recur. ____

7. After Loretta connects her panicky states to being alone and how she felt reassured by your availability, you should

A. Discuss the intolerance of aloneness as a symptom of BPD and how it handicaps relationships. ____
B. Offer to help her develop alternative ways to manage her crises because you are not reliably available. ____
C. Encourage her to call *before* such crises because only then can you help prevent their escalation. ____
D. Praise her for uncovering the basic problem with being alone and assure her that it can change. ____
E. Discuss alternative ways to manage her aloneness. ____

Discussion

1. In response to Loretta's wish to be treated for her depression and anxiety, you should

    (see "Basic Therapeutic Approach" in Chapter 2 and "How to Disclose" in Chapter 3)

    A. Agree to prioritize these symptoms. [3] (This will encourage unrealistic hopes for symptom relief and ignore the more central issue of her interpersonal crises.)

    B. Tell her that she has BPD and this explains her symptoms. [2] (Even if Loretta accepts your diagnosis of BPD and its causal role in her anxiety and depression, this approach is too authoritative, requires more diagnostic assessment, does not involve her as a collaborator, and is too totalitarian [does not encourage more partialed out explanation].)

    C. Ask her to review the criteria for BPD, noting that it might explain her symptoms. [1] (Yes, this involves her and increases her self-awareness. When the BPD diagnosis is confirmed, psychoeducation should then be given.)

2. In response to Loretta's insomnia and panic attacks, you should

    (see "Good Psychiatric Management Theory: Interpersonal Hypersensitivity" and "Basic Therapeutic Approach" in Chapter 2; Chapter 5; and "General Principles" in Chapter 6)

    A. Begin a suicide risk assessment. [3] (It is good to be active and responsive, but this is an overreaction. You want to model being thoughtful and curious. You might inquire about what "feeling unsafe" means. The borderline patient should introduce the issue of suicidality, not the treaters.)

    B. Inquire whether these symptoms are related to problems with her boyfriend. [1] (Whenever anxiety [or depression] is exacerbated, an interpersonal stress is very likely. She's already acknowledged this in her first session.)

    C. Express concern and invite her to contact you before her anxiety escalates. [3] (This is fine if you are a Dialectical Behavior Therapy [DBT]–based or a skill-based clinician; otherwise, to do this invites a helpless patient–rescuer treater dyad and may prove undesirably burdensome. That is not helpful or realistic.)

D. Ask whether there is any way you could help. **[2]** (This is okay but should follow inquiries into the sources of her insomnia and panic symptoms.)

E. Express concern about whether the session with you had worsened these symptoms. **[2]** (This is definitely a good consideration, i.e., is the patient regressing in response to your caregiving? Still, it is probably premature to raise this issue in the second session. At this point, situational causes should be explored. If these symptoms continue to worsen, or even not get better in the next few months, it would certainly be wise to raise this question.)

F. Review possible medication changes. **[3]** (There may come a time for this, but medications are a secondary strategy. You don't want Loretta to think that medications are likely to solve her symptoms. You do want her to consider the psychological and social sources of her symptoms. Through those considerations, the patient might take control of her symptoms.)

3. When Loretta asks whether she might call you if she needs to, you should

(see "Good Psychiatric Management Theory: Interpersonal Hypersensitivity" and "Basic Therapeutic Approach" in Chapter 2 and "Intersession Availability" in Chapter 4)

A. Discourage her from calling you. **[3]** (This response will tell the patient that you fear being unnecessarily called or that you do not want to be involved in her crises. Such fears may or may not be justified but should be assessed by first asking under what circumstances she might "need" to talk with you—see responses B and D for this discussion.)

B. Inquire how she hopes talking with you could be helpful. **[1]** (This is a good way to invite discussion of the basic underlying issues of loneliness, lack of supports, and so forth.)

C. Encourage her to use the local crisis hotline. **[2]** (This advice is not necessarily harmful, but it will likely feel like a rejection. It is inconsistent with developing the "real" side of your interpersonal connection [i.e., the dyadic model] that is itself therapeutic. It does not communicate your wish to be helpful, and it will discourage her from trusting or depending on you—which would be positive developments for borderline patients.)

D. Ask her to describe circumstances where she might "need" to call you. **[1]** (Yes, this is essential.)

E. Note that she cannot count on your always being available, and discuss other ways that she can manage crises. [2] (This is safe and will be good enough for most BPD patients. However, this approach should be used only after discussing what she "needs," i.e., responses B and D for this discussion. Moreover, it may discourage the one or two calls that can bring the issue of aloneness and the need for a caring other into focus.)

4. In response to Loretta's highly distressed 11:30 call, you should

(see Chapter 4)

A. Empathize with her distress. [1] (Essential.)
B. Ask what she and her boyfriend fought about. [3] (She might insist on telling you, but this is not the occasion to invite a detailed description of the situational stresses. This chain analysis is best reserved for the next session.)
C. Encourage her to breathe deeply and count to 100 when she has such episodes of panic. [3] (This is generally helpful advice but not after the episode and not in a late-night call. Notably, she seemed to have gained relief by your answering her call and listening to her problems. That is a more important observation to be highlighted for discussion in subsequent sessions.)
D. Apologetically tell her that you were asleep, and offer her an additional appointment in the morning. [2] (It is good to acknowledge that your helpfulness is handicapped by having been asleep, and by offering to see her in the morning, you convey concern. However, introducing this issue too abruptly may aggravate her guilt or seem rejecting. This consideration should await discussion within scheduled sessions.)

5. When Loretta calls again several hours later saying "I don't know whether I can go on like this," you should

(see "Basic Therapeutic Approach" in Chapter 2; "Setting the Framework" in Chapter 4; and "Common Problems" in Chapter 5):

A. Tell her to develop a safety plan. [2] (React yes, but this is overreactive. Don't assume her comment is a suicide threat. It is more likely a bid for caregiving. Assessing whether she is suicidal is essential, but unless there is confirmation, dwelling too much on her safety will lengthen the call and might reinforce her use of suicidality as the way to gain care.)

B. Ask what her concern with "going on" refers to. [1] (Yes, this encourages Loretta to think. It could refer to her partnership with her boyfriend or to her overall life, or even to her therapy. The implications of each option are quite different. This inquiry focuses her on the interpersonal context that is likely to be causal.)

C. Encourage her to seek help at an emergency department. [3] (Again, you don't know if she's suicidal, and, if she were, this option shouldn't be introduced until other alternatives—thinking about the source of her distress—are considered.)

D. Ask whether you had failed to be helpful in the prior call. [2] (This is a very good question to consider, but it's too exploratory. At present, she needs to be stabilized, and you want to go back to sleep.)

E. Inquire whether she has tried to reach her boyfriend. [2] (This is a reasonable question. However, it may invite a prolonged discussion about the situational stressors. Your goals are to calm her, assure safety, and go back to sleep.)

F. Reassure her that you are not angry and that you plan to work with her for as long as it takes. [3] (The reassurance is fine, but the promise for the future is overreactive and will reinforce her calling you. Such a promissory response probably indicates a failure to own your distaste for being repeatedly awakened. You need to be a real person for Loretta, and a professional.)

6. In the next session, when Loretta describes her recurrent crises with Carl, you should

(see "Basic Therapeutic Approach" in Chapter 2)

A. Listen carefully and encourage her to talk more about this issue [3] (It is an important issue, but the call itself is the primary issue that needs attention.)

B. Interrupt her discussion of the relationship and ask her to discuss what occurred during the telephone call. [1] (It is easy not to do this. But not asking implies that the call was not a significant event. That encourages more calls and misses an important opportunity to discuss the role you played [see response D for this discussion] and the issues of intersession contacts such as expectations, roles, and safety planning.)

C. Note how the hostile dependent relationship with Carl is similar to what she has described with her parents. [2] (This is a valuable observation but secondary to the focus on the here-and-now situation posed by the telephone call.)

D. Ask her whether calling you had been helpful and, if so, why. **[1]** (This is a very important bridge into issues of loneliness, rescue fantasies, idealization, the realities of your limits, and considerations of alternative safety plans.)

E. Indicate that having your sleep disrupted was irritating but that you were also glad to be helpful. **[2]** (Again, this is an important message, but Loretta is unlikely to be able to process your irritation. This response should be introduced when the alliance is stronger.)

F. Consider other ways to deal with this should the situation recur. **[1]** (This is always a good issue—not to be rejecting but to underscore the realities of your limitations.)

7. After Loretta connects her panicky states to being alone and says she felt reassured by your availability, you should

   (see "Good Psychiatric Management Theory: Interpersonal Hypersensitivity" and "Basic Therapeutic Approach" in Chapter 2 and "Impending Self-Endangering Behaviors" and "The Aftermath of Self-Endangering Behaviors" in Chapter 5)

   A. Discuss the intolerance of aloneness as a symptom of BPD and how it handicaps relationships. **[1]** (People feel more in control if able to explain their otherwise inchoate experiences. This discussion sets the stage for examining ways to limit their recurrence.)

   B. Offer to help her develop alternative ways to manage her crises because you are not reliably available. **[2]** (Discussing alternatives is good, but the primary issue should be managing rejection and aloneness, not her crises per se.)

   C. Encourage her to call *before* such crises because only then can you help prevent their escalation. **[2]** (This approach is encouraged within the DBT model. Its value within the GPM model would rest on talking meaningfully about impending fears of rejection and aloneness.)

   D. Praise her for uncovering the basic problem with being alone and assure her that it can change. **[1]** (Yes, she has reflected on her experience, disclosed her observations, and taken a big step toward self-awareness. A real insight!)

   E. Discuss alternative ways to manage her aloneness. **[1]** (Yes, you want to convert the discussion away from preventing suicide into improving her life outside treatment; namely, getting caring partners into her life.)

Case 3, April: Somatization and Alliance Building

Illustrating Chapters 2, 4, and 6

This vignette illustrates the need to discuss goals and roles, assess the alliance, and provide psychoeducation. It also illustrates the treater's persistent efforts to move a patient's search for medication relief of symptoms into a discussion of psychosocial contributions to her pain and distress.

Case Vignette

April is referred to you by her primary care physician, who has concluded that she has BPD and requires psychiatric care. She presents as a slightly unkempt, pleasant, and soft-spoken overweight 34-year-old woman. She has a long history of depression, anxiety, somatic complaints, and severe self-mutilation—making multiple, and at times deep, cuts in her forearms and legs. She complains of chronic depression that can make it difficult for her to get out of bed and of anxiety so severe that it has caused her to "feel frozen." She has a history of alcohol abuse but has been abstinent for 1 month. She is 70 pounds overweight and has a history of binge eating, particularly during the evening. On the basis of her self-harm, help-seeking, affective instability, and impulsivity, you feel confident of the BPD diagnosis.

April also reports complicated medical problems (i.e., chronic pain from arthritis, fibromyalgia, migraines, asthma, and diabetes). She has been treated with various types and doses of medications, including opiates. She is focused on how much pain she is in and immediately requests that you refer her to specialists for treatment of her migraines and painful menses.

She has a strong academic record but has never been able to hold a job for more than 6 months and has remained financially dependent on her family. She has few friends. April recently began attending business school. This involved relocating from living with her parents to an apartment with several roommates. "My parents," she says, "especially my mother, are upset about the costs."

At the end of this session, you feel certain of the borderline diagnosis and have a clearer picture of April's problems. [**Decision Point 1**] You also feel a bit overwhelmed by the complexity of her medical and medication history. When you schedule her return, you ask her to prepare a medical/medication summary and bring it to her next meeting.

At her return visit, a week later, she complains of worsening depression and that she is feeling more hopeless about her life. She says that she has been unable to work on the medical/medication summary, explaining that fights with her mother preoccupy her. She feels that her mother has become less and less understanding ever since she decided to return to school. That, she says, is why she moved into her current apartment. Although she does not appear depressed, she insists that if she does not receive an antidepressant, she will not be able to function. She notes that sertraline has been helpful in the past. [**Decision Point 2**] You set up a third appointment, this time for a half-hour, with the understanding that she will have sent you her medical/medication history.

She returns for her third visit (still without having sent the medical/medication history), stating that her urges to harm herself have increased and that she is thinking more frequently about cutting herself again. These urges, she says, have become more intense as her most recent prior wounds in her forearms have healed. She then describes increased conflict with one of her roommates, who she insists has been unfriendly to her since she moved in. [**Decision Point 3**] When you ask about the medical/medication summary, she apologetically says that she has made no progress. At the end of this session, she appears angry. When you ask about this, she says "you're not being very helpful." You tell her that you fear she's right and set up another half-hour appointment.

April sends you a carefully detailed medical/medication history but then arrives 15 minutes late for her next visit. She explains that she was late because she had not been able to get out of bed, adding that she had not slept more than a few hours each night for several days because of severe fibromyalgia. She believes that the pain has worsened since she began walking 20 minutes per day to try to get in shape. You express appreciation for her exercise and then ask her about the status of her fights with her mother and her roommate. She doesn't respond to this, going on to say that she finds it almost impossible to concentrate on her schoolwork and then says that she needs narcotics for her muscle and joint pain, noting they have been very helpful in the past. You confirm this from her summary sheet, but, trying to end the visit on time, you say that you will need to discuss this further. She immediately looks angry and asserts that "you do not understand my pain." [**Decision Point 4**]

April returns for a follow-up hour-long appointment several days later. She appears irritated and says, "I wonder whether you are really interested in treating me?" You reassure her that you are. She then complains that her pain remains severe, that she is not sleeping, and that you have not prescribed the medications she has been telling you she needs. She again insists that she needs a narcotic for her pain, adding that she has cut herself superficially on her right forearm. She says that sometimes she thinks that she would be better off dead. [**Decision Point 5**]

You tell her that you too are concerned with your failure to have helped her. You talk to her about how her symptoms are rarely responsive to medications but usually can be relieved by decreasing stress. She doesn't seem to be placated by this, complaining that "doctors should try to make their patients feel better." Feeling somewhat defeated, you tell her that she might be helped by getting consultation and added support from a pain clinic. She agrees to this. You also decide that maybe a trial of a selective serotonin reuptake inhibitor would buy time while you work to address her stressors. She seems pleased by this. You further suggest that maybe you could talk with her mother to help decrease the stress that comes from that part of her life.

April is a particularly difficult patient with whom it will be hard to develop an alliance without enacting some supportive interventions that are not likely to be effective, such as giving her some medications. It will probably be useful, if feasible, to involve her mother. Her mother doesn't seem likely to be any more psychologically minded than is April, but that needs to be evaluated. Even if her mother is not allied with treatment goals, April will appreciate that you are actively doing things to help her. Meeting with the mother will help you better understand their fights—or the problems they both have with her becoming independent. April also might get support from involvement in a group; perhaps a pain or other medically based group.

Decision Points: Alternative Responses

(1 = will be helpful, 2 = possibly helpful, continuing reservations, 3 = not helpful—or even harmful)
See next subsection for discussion.

1. At the end of this first session, you have the impression that

    A. April's current help-seeking is probably triggered by the anxieties of leaving home and attending school. ___
    B. It will be a gradual process taking months, or possibly years, for her somatic preoccupations to recede. ___
    C. April's somatic preoccupations are symptomatic of underlying emptiness and unmet dependency needs. ___
    D. The first priority will be to wean her from pain medications. ___
    E. The first priority will be to sort out goals and roles. ___
    F. April's treatment will require intensive individual psychotherapy. ___

2. In response to April's request for sertraline for her depression, you should

    A. Ask her more about her experience of feeling depressed and inquire about neurovegetative symptoms. ___
    B. Ask whether her recent difficulties with her mother might be contributing to the way she is feeling. ___
    C. Offer to prescribe sertraline to facilitate alliance building. ___
    D. Agree that antidepressants might be helpful but indicate that they are adjunctive and unlikely to have major benefits for her. ___
    E. Advise the patient that the requested summary of her medical/medication history is needed before making decisions about medication change. ___

3. When April returns with escalating impulses to self-harm, you should

A. Express serious concern about the urges and introduce the possibility of hospitalization. ___

B. Express concern about the patient's self-destructive urges but then move on to other topics lest you reinforce their use as a "cry for help." ___

C. Explore whether her renewed urges to self-injure are related to the conflict with her roommate or other stressful events. ___

D. Discuss whether the self-destructive urges have an addictive quality and might respond to naltrexone. ___

4. In response to April's neglected homework, lateness, increased physical pain, and apparent anger, you should

A. Tell the patient that because of her lateness, insufficient time is available to adequately address her pain. ___ .

B. Schedule a 1-hour follow-up appointment for as soon as reasonable. ___

C. Offer the patient a prescription for oxycodone. ___

D. Acknowledge her unhappiness with you and say that this needs to be discussed in her next appointment. ___

5. In response to April's escalating pain and questions about your value, you should

A. Take a careful history of her pain and its relation to stress. ___

B. Tell the patient that you will not prescribe narcotics for her because you are concerned about the possible harm from opioids for someone who drinks alcohol and because you are concerned that she may not use opioids as prescribed. ___

C. Express concern for her continued pain but then ask whether her pain and self-laceration are the result of her current stressors. ___

D. Point out that you too are troubled about how the treatment has evolved and encourage her to discuss that. ___

E. Note how each of your meetings has been associated with an acute and changing symptom for which she has requested medications, and in each instance you have responded by wanting to examine how these symptoms relate to her stressful life situations. ___

F. Provide psychoeducation about her disorder and stress that her symptoms (such as depression, anxiety, or self-harm) are only weakly affected by medications but often can be relieved by changing the life situations that prompt them—especially learning to cope with interpersonal problems in new ways. ___

Discussion

1. At the end of this first session, you have the impression that

   (see "Basic Therapeutic Approach" in Chapter 2; "Setting the Framework" and "Common Problems" in Chapter 4; and "General Principles" and "Building an Alliance" in Chapter 6)

   A. April's current help-seeking is probably triggered by the anxieties of leaving home and attending school. [1] (Insofar as April had BPD, this is a critically important consideration. April will not volunteer this insight even if she is aware of it. By knowing this, you will become more comfortable being cautious about medications. By helping her accept this, you will help her rely less on somatic complaints and develop common goals more readily.)

   B. It will be a gradual process taking months, or possibly years, for her somatic preoccupations to recede. [1] (Getting impatient or trying to set limits on her somatic complaints will be predictable temptations, but these are deeply entrenched help-seeking patterns that may with time [more awareness of feeling and of separation anxieties and more success] become more dystonic.)

   C. April's somatic preoccupations are symptomatic of underlying emptiness and unmet dependency needs. [1] (While this interpretation seems speculative, it is buttressed by noting her hostile dependent relationship with her mother and her failure to achieve vocational stability or financial independence despite apparent intellectual aptitude, and above all by understanding the interpersonal basis for the borderline diagnosis.)

   D. The first priority will be to wean her from pain medications. [3] (Her preoccupation with medications may force their management into being the primary focus, but whether, within this focus, weaning her from the pain medicines is a realistic first goal is unlikely. A careful assessment, with her collaboration, of the effects of prior pain medications, including her compliance, is needed. Giving April the homework writing task to address this is a very good first step in this process.)

   E. The first priority will be to sort out goals and roles. [1] (Yes, April seems interested in using you as a pain reliever. You need to educate her—expressing regrets—about the modest benefits she can probably expect from medications. You also need to see whether she can accept your goal to examine the psychosocial sources of her depression and pain and other somatic complaints.)

F. April's treatment will require intensive individual psychotherapy. [3] (April is a very difficult patient in part because she does not "psychologize" her inner problems; she "somatizes" them. It will be a very significant achievement to connect her somatic complaints to situational precipitants and from there to help her accept feelings. Achieving these improvements will probably be accompanied by reduced medical help-seeking and reduced medication dependency. At that point, perhaps, some form of psychotherapy might be beneficial.)

2. In response to April's request for sertraline for her depression, you should

(see "Good Psychiatric Management Theory: Interpersonal Hypersensitivity" and "Basic Therapeutic Approach" in Chapter 2; "Common Problems" in Chapter 4; and "General Principles," "Building an Alliance," and "Comorbidities" in Chapter 6)

A. Ask her more about her experience of feeling depressed and inquire about neurovegetative symptoms. [3] (The pursuit of her symptom complaint may be worthwhile if you are preparing to prescribe. At this point in this case, however, this response will reinforce her use of you as a pain reliever and avoid the tasks of involving her as a responsible collaborator in addressing psychosocial issues.)

B. Ask whether her recent difficulties with her mother might be contributing to the way she is feeling. [1] (This encourages the patient to connect her symptoms to her situation; most notably, to interpersonal events. She would not be expected to see such a connection at this point, but you are introducing her to looking for antecedent causes.)

C. Offer to prescribe sertraline to facilitate alliance building. [3] (She may welcome this, but it is a precedent that will reinforce the false expectation that negative affective states can be readily addressed with pharmacotherapy and that this is what she should expect from you. Her "alliance" will now become based on you as likeable and helpful, i.e., "a pain reliever," but without agreeing about your roles and goals and not on you and her as collaborating partners.)

D. Agree that antidepressants might be helpful but indicate that they are adjunctive and unlikely to have major benefits for her. [1] (This helps the patient feel that you are concerned about her symptoms but that her depression is unlikely to respond to antidepressants. It also indicates that you and she need to be careful and cautious about her prescriptions.)

E. Advise the patient that the requested summary of her medical/medication history is needed before making decisions about medication change. [1] (This requires April to become active in her treatment, and it underscores the need to think carefully before acting.)

3. When April returns with escalating impulses to self-harm, you should

(see "Good Psychiatric Management Theory: Interpersonal Hypersensitivity" in Chapter 2, "Impending Self-Endangering Behaviors" in Chapter 5, and "General Principles" in Chapter 6)

A. Express serious concern about the urges and introduce the possibility of hospitalization. [3] (Expressing concern is good, but introducing the issue of hospitalization at this point is premature and potentially harmful. Assessment of risk is required. Cutting is not usually dangerous. April needs to become involved in self-examination and self-care. Hospitalization might be welcomed as a flight from both. This response also will encourage the impression that self-injury offers a way to escape her life situation and personal accountability and that you are unable to work with her on changing her use of this behavior.)

B. Express concern about the patient's self-destructive urges but then move on to other topics lest you reinforce their use as a "cry for help." [3] (The rationale might be correct, but this response will leave the patient feeling invalidated and dismissed by you.)

C. Explore whether her renewed urges to self-injure are related to the conflict with her roommate or other stressful events. [1] (This again shows the patient that you are interested in her symptoms and their relation to situational stress—notably, interpersonal events. What may be of greater significance than the roommate are the larger life changes, as noted earlier, of having moved out of home and the increased fights with her mother. These are major shifts in April's holding environment.)

D. Discuss whether the self-destructive urges have an addictive quality and might respond to naltrexone. [3] (This inquiry is not responsive to the psychosocial context of these urges, including the still very insecure alliance with you. Consideration of initiating naltrexone will only reinforce her use of you as an analgesic and her failure to take an active role in self-care. Naltrexone, or any other medication, is also unlikely to reduce her self-harm.)

4. In response to April's neglected homework, lateness, increased physical pain, and apparent anger, you should

   (see "Basic Therapeutic Approach" in Chapter 2 and "Setting the Framework" in Chapter 4)

   A. Tell the patient that because of her lateness, insufficient time is available to adequately address her pain. [2] (This limit may be realistic and is almost certainly useful, but it should be made with apologies, to diminish her feeling cruelly mistreated and angry.)
   B. Schedule a 1-hour follow-up appointment for as soon as reasonable. [1] (The 1-hour follow-up in the near future is warranted in view of her evident anger and the ongoing conflicts about roles and goals. Unfortunately, it also may reinforce getting attention through dysfunction, but this treatment is unlikely to last unless you add supportive actions that will indicate concern.)
   C. Offer the patient a prescription for oxycodone. [3] (Prescribing a potentially addictive medication to a patient who is late, with multiple and changing symptoms, with little alliance, and in the absence of an extended discussion is dangerous.)
   D. Acknowledge her unhappiness with you and say that this needs to be discussed in her next appointment. [1] (Yes, there has been a growing schism between her wants and your services. A serious discussion about this disparity and whether it can be resolved is needed.)

5. In response to April's escalating pain and questions about your value, you should

   (see "Basic Therapeutic Approach" in Chapter 2)

   A. Take a careful history of her pain and its relation to stress. [3] (This information gathering is a necessary prelude to decisions about treating her pain, but it overlooks the more pressing issues concerning her complaints about you and the clearly disparate goals evident within your sessions.)
   B. Tell the patient that you will not prescribe narcotics for her because you are concerned about the possible harm from opioids for someone who drinks alcohol and because you are concerned that she may not use opioids as prescribed. [3] (This response to her specific requests will aggravate her alienation. Moreover, it is the larger problems within the treatment that need attention.)
   C. Express concern for her continued pain but then ask whether her pain and self-laceration are the result of her current stressors. [2]

(This response complements response A for this discussion. It validates your concern for April's pain and encourages her to make connections to her current situation. By itself, however, it would not address the relation of her escalating pain to the problems she is having with her treater.)

D. Point out that you too are troubled about how the treatment has evolved and encourage her to discuss that. [1] (Yes, her symptoms are worsening, not getting better. The problem in the therapeutic alliance needs to be the first priority.)

E. Note how each of your meetings has been associated with an acute and changing symptom for which she has requested medications, and in each instance you have responded by wanting to examine how these symptoms relate to her stressful life situations. [1] (This is a helpful summary of the pattern that has developed in these initial sessions. She then should be invited to discuss this, getting into the apparent disparity of her hopes and your services. Whether and how this can be resolved are necessary questions to be addressed.)

F. Provide psychoeducation about her disorder and stress that her symptoms (such as depression, anxiety, or self-harm) are only weakly affected by medications but often can be relieved by changing the life situations that prompt them—especially learning to cope with interpersonal problems in new ways. [1] (Psychoeducation and clarification of roles and goals are essential and probably overdue. There is a good chance that April will not want what you have to offer. There is a greater risk, however, of doing her harm by not addressing her reliance on medications or, worse, by giving her medications that have never helped.)

Case 4, Laura: Hospitalization and Dependency

Illustrating Chapters 2, 4, and 5

Escalating self-harm and repeated hospitalizations lead to a change in treaters. The patient quickly connects to the new treater, who manages to build an alliance while interrupting her regressive reactions to his absence. This case illustrates the skills required to interrupt a harmfully repeated pattern of hospitalizations but ends with the equally formidable challenge of helping the patient get on with developing a satisfactory life.

Case Vignette

Laura, a 25-year-old woman with BPD, is now hospitalized for the eighth time in 2 years. Both the psychotherapist and the psychiatrist who have worked with her during this time informed the patient and the inpatient case manager that they are no longer willing to work with Laura given her increase in both self-harming and suicidal behaviors over time. [**Decision Point 1**] You are called to consult on her treatment and explore the possibility of starting as her new psychiatrist. [**Decision Point 2**]

Laura is an anxious, overweight, baby-faced woman who appears both sullen and fearful. She softly explains that she has had a long history of self-harming since age 16, when her parents began to have marital problems. You gently ask her to speak up because you're having trouble hearing her. With a brief smile, she complies. She then described that she cut herself to relieve emotional pain when she was anxious or sad about her parents' situation but never told them how she felt. Her parents eventually found out about her cutting through the school counselor, and they banded together to help her get treatment. She liked the treater, a social worker, and her cutting decreased. However, when Laura left home to start college, she began cutting more frequently and eventually began overdosing on medications. Laura reports that in subsequent years, she increasingly didn't care if she lived, because she was often struggling with sadness or anxiety and with believing she was unlovable and bad. Her overdoses were intended "to make those feelings go away." These overdoses have involved 10–15 tablets of Prozac, which made her feel ill but which she knew would not kill her. In response to these overdoses, she had been hospitalized and received medication changes.

Laura's previous therapist and psychiatrist both reported that when Laura was upset, she engaged in reckless binge drinking. When they expressed frustration about this, she felt "misunderstood." Moreover, she would not show up for appointments when she was most distressed and would not call before taking her self-harming or suicidal actions. [**Decision Point 3**]

You begin a combined psychopharmacology and psychotherapy weekly treatment with Laura. Although she missed some appointments, the treatment generally went well. Laura was active and disclosing, and you found her interesting and thoughtful. Laura's attendance improved, and she used e-mail or texting to cancel or alter appointments. She had begun working part time as a dog walker. Three months into the treatment, you went away for a meeting. Laura refused to see the covering doctor and cut herself. She sent you an e-mail that she really needs to talk and can't be safe without you. [**Decision Point 4**]

In the session after you return, you discuss with Laura the events that happened when you were away. In this discussion, Laura says, "I depend on you so heavily that I became panicked in your absence and I could not imagine that anyone else would be able to help me." Emphasizing her safety, you reiterate that she needs to be able to see a covering treater when you are away. Laura says, "Then just put me in a hospital" and, sobbing, runs out of the office. [**Decision Point 5**]

Laura ends up going to the emergency department and accepts voluntary admission into the hospital. She does not self-harm or overdose before her admission. You visit her in the hospital. [**Decision Point 6**]

Over the next 6 months, Laura's course is one of inconsistent improvements, but she failed to return to her part-time work as a dog walker. Gradually she comes to trust your good intentions, the use of alcohol stops altogether, and her self-harm fades away. Suicidal ideation is persistent, but you no longer worry about her taking overdoses. She regresses when you are away (goes to bed, overeats) and still does not contact the covering doctor, but she has had no more hospitalizations. She is stable but seems to hold her parents hostage via her disability and dependency. She talks about that, but you worry whether she's going to "get a life."

Decision Points: Alternative Responses

(1 = will be helpful, 2 = possibly helpful, continuing reservations, 3 = not helpful—or even harmful)

See next subsection for discussion.

1. Laura's inpatient case manager should respond to the prior treaters' announced intention to terminate their involvement by

   A. Urging them to reconsider because Laura's unresponsiveness isn't their fault. ___
   B. Advising Laura that her continued self-destructiveness signals a treatment that hasn't been effective. ___
   C. Assessing whether Laura's escalating self-harm is a result of the prior treatment. ___

2. In assessing whether to treat Laura, you should

   A. Ask Laura to sign a written contract that she will not self-harm or kill herself. ___
   B. Ask her prior clinicians whether she's treatable. ___
   C. Assess dangerousness, differentiating nonlethal from true suicidal intention. ___
   D. First attain a history of the patient's childhood to understand the developmental sources of her suicidality. ___

3. After assessing Laura's suicidality, you should

   A. Discuss how Laura can help herself when she is in situations or emotional states that lead her to self-harm or overdose. ___
   B. Insist on being paged when she is going to self-harm or overdose. ___
   C. Indicate that you need to discuss what leads her to self-harm or overdose. ___

    D. Ask Laura whether her self-destructive impulses and actions were related to experiences of loneliness or rejection. ___

    E. Tell her that the safest plan is for her to go to the emergency department when suicidal. ___

    F. Express concerns about alcohol use as a risk factor. ___

    G. Explore why she felt misunderstood by her prior treaters' reactions and why she didn't call them before her self-destructive acts. ___

4. In response to Laura's desperate e-mail, you should

    A. Call Laura and insist that she see the covering doctor. ___

    B. Call the covering doctor and encourage him or her to contact Laura about her safety. ___

    C. Call 911 and have her hospitalized. ___

    D. E-mail Laura and let her know you're concerned and that you want to discuss this more on your return, but in the meantime, she needs to use either the covering physician or emergency services. ___

5. When Laura runs out of your office, you should

    A. Call the police and have her hospitalized. ___

    B. Call after her to come back, assuring her that you will discuss whether hospitalization is needed. ___

    C. Not pursue her, but leave her a message that you are troubled by the way the session ended and that you want her either to go to the emergency department or to respond to your message. ___

6. When you meet with Laura in the hospital, you should

    A. Ask Laura to detail what happened before the self-harm event while you were away and before her abrupt departure from your office. ___

    B. Invoke a split treatment so that another physician is managing the medications while you continue the therapy. ___

    C. Explore her apparent dependency on you. ___

    D. Discuss your dilemma about hospitalization—that is, that it makes her safe but may become (or already has become) regressive and life-interfering. Note that "our failure" (thereby including yourself as part of the problem) to have a constructive conversation about this in your office reflects the fragility of this treatment. ___

    E. Be concerned about possible liability and seek forensic
       advice. ___

    F. Suggest that she tell her family about what happened. ___

Discussion

1. Laura's inpatient case manager should respond to the prior treaters' announced intention to terminate their involvement by

   (see "Basic Therapeutic Approach" in Chapter 2; "Setting the Framework" in Chapter 4; and Chapter 5)

   A. Urging them to reconsider because Laura's unresponsiveness isn't their fault. [3] (It may well not be their fault, but Laura's 2-year course testifies to a failed treatment and their intention to terminate testifies to having exhausted either their skills or their patience.)

   B. Advising Laura that her continued self-destructiveness signals a treatment that hasn't been effective. [1] (Yes, she should be reoriented toward expecting change and proactively making efforts to establish a better treatment.)

   C. Assessing whether Laura's escalating self-harm is a result of the prior treatment. [1] (Yes, knowledge about both the usual course of improvement and that many treaters are ill informed about how to treat BPD should definitely raise this question. In this case, the expected need for hospitalization may reflect a treatment that was overreactive and didn't involve Laura as a collaborator. How you proceed depends on the answer to this question.)

2. In assessing whether to treat Laura, you should

   (see Chapters 2 and 5)

   A. Ask Laura to sign a written contract that she will not self-harm or kill herself. [3] (A written contract for safety might be helpful, but it cannot replace a collaboration-generating discussion about managing self-destructive tendencies. Contracting for safety is usually not effective with borderline patients, whose states of mind [and risk] can change quickly and dramatically. Understanding what prompts Laura's pattern of self-harming or suicidal tendencies is critical for safety planning and as an alliance-building intervention when done collaboratively with the patient.)

B. Ask her prior clinicians whether she's treatable. [2] (Prior treaters can be instructive, but they usually cannot be expected to be good judges of whether a patient is treatable. You yourself need to judge whether you can offer effective interventions for this patient. Understanding the problems that have occurred in prior treatments and how prior treatment relationships affected Laura's self-endangering behaviors will help you anticipate similar problems and then proactively discuss how you and the patient might better address these issues.)

C. Assess dangerousness, differentiating nonlethal from true suicidal intention. [1] (This is an essential first step in deciding whether and how—i.e., under what level of care—you can treat Laura.)

D. First attain a history of the patient's childhood to understand the developmental sources of her suicidality. [3] (While appreciating that developmental factors influence suicidality, this is often not easily accomplished. Assessing the here-and-now risk for life-endangering behaviors is the necessary and sufficient priority.)

3. After assessing Laura's suicidality, you should

(see Chapters 2 and 5)

A. Discuss how Laura can help herself when she is in situations or emotional states that lead her to self-harm or overdose. [1] (A problem-solving effort emphasizing agency to manage safety will be valuable. Laura probably will be resistant, and this then becomes the central consideration.)

B. Insist on being paged when she is going to self-harm or overdose. [3] (This option may encourage unrealistic expectations of your availability. It is important for Laura to have a plan for when you are unavailable. Laura needs to consider what she believes would help and how she might access it. If she needs to talk to someone, discuss her options, including yourself, while being clear that she cannot depend on your availability.)

C. Indicate that you need to discuss what leads her to self-harm or overdose. [1] (This is definitely a good idea. Underscore the message that self-harm and suicidality are reactions to life events—usually, interpersonal ones.)

D. Ask Laura whether her self-destructive impulses and actions were related to experiences of loneliness or rejection. [1] (Understanding the significance of these interpersonal experiences as triggers

is a big first step toward improving their avoidance and management. It moves her understanding of self-harm away from reactions to unwanted feelings to reactions that have meaning in her
internal life and outside situations.)

E. Tell her that the safest plan is for her to go to the emergency department when suicidal. [2] (This is helpful when the patient can
manage this on her own. Its downsides are 1) it may be inter-
preted as your lack of concern, and 2) it may result in an unnecessary hospitalization by others that will reinforce its use as an
avoidance strategy.)

F. Express concerns about alcohol use as a risk factor. [1] (Laura
should be educated about how alcohol use increases disinhibition
and impulsivity.)

G. Explore why she felt misunderstood by her prior treaters' reactions and why she didn't call them before her self-destructive acts.
[1] (Ask whether this might recur with you. Making these issues
explicit helps anticipate their recurrence and sets the stage for a
problem-solving discussion.)

4. In response to Laura's desperate e-mail, you should

*(see "Good Psychiatric Management Theory: Interpersonal Hy-
persensitivity" and "Basic Therapeutic Approach" in Chapter 2
and Chapters 4 and 5)*

A. Call Laura and insist that she see the covering doctor. [3] (By calling her, you make yourself available and undermine the message
that she needs to use the covering doctor—or otherwise take care
of herself in your absence. You may need to remind yourself that
Laura's cutting [and even her overdoses] have never been dangerous.)

B. Call the covering doctor and encourage him or her to contact
Laura about her safety. [2] (This conveys concern while maintain-
ing a limit around your absences. Still, the reliance on the initiative of the covering doctor does not require that Laura take an
active role in her own safety.)

C. Call 911 and have her hospitalized. [3] (This is overreactive. This
assumes that she is at risk despite no history of dangerousness.
Moreover, the containment given by being hospitalized may have
already become a "bad habit"—a way for Laura to relieve her distress without active participation or learning.)

D. E-mail Laura and let her know that you're concerned and want to discuss this more on your return, but that in the meantime, she needs to use either the covering physician or emergency services. [1] (It is important to communicate that you intend to resume work with her while helping her be responsible for her own safety by use of the prescribed resources. On returning, establish that you will not be available for e-mails while away.)

5. When Laura runs out of your office, you should

(see "Basic Therapeutic Approach" in Chapter 2 and Chapter 5)

A. Call the police and have her hospitalized. [3] (Although it is prudent not to ignore possible self-endangerment, hospitalization is probably overreactive. It would, in any event, be another failure to involve her in her own safety. Past "suicide attempts" have been communicative "cries for help.")

B. Call after her to come back, assuring her that you will discuss whether hospitalization is needed. [2] (This reaction validates your concern for her safety and might interrupt her flight. If she returns, the discussion should include whether hospitalization is needed and its potential downside. This discussion may make you late for other responsibilities but should take precedence. It should not, however, be so prolonged as to be too gratifying. Moreover, you should not resume a psychotherapy-like discussion of the interpersonal dynamics.)

C. Don't pursue her, but leave her a message that you are troubled by the way the session ended and that you want her either to go to the emergency department or to respond to your message. [1] (Communicating concern and an expectation that she can manage her own safety is optimal. Assessing and managing risk without hospitalization have the advantage of emphasizing the importance of internal controls, i.e., her agency. This response also emphasizes the role of dialogue as the optimal management strategy for emotional and interpersonal problems.)

6. When you meet with Laura in the hospital, you should

(see "Good Psychiatric Management Theory: Interpersonal Hypersensitivity" and "How Change Occurs" in Chapter 2, Chapter 5, and "Rationale" and "Selecting Another Modality" in Chapter 7, "Split Treatments")

A. Ask Laura to detail what happened before the self-harm event while you were away and then before her departure from your office. [1] (A collaborative chain analysis of the emotional and interpersonal factors leading to acts of self-harm, suicidality, or angry flights is essential for increasing self-awareness and safety planning for the future. If possible, Laura should have been encouraged to do this "homework" before your visit. Such analyses invest the patient with some responsibility, highlight moments when alternative actions were possible, and convey your belief in his or her capacity to manage.).

B. Invoke a split treatment so that another physician is managing the medications while you continue the therapy. [2] (Because Laura had difficulty managing your time away and seeing a clinician with whom she was unfamiliar, it might be helpful to establish a split treatment. It also may diminish the idealization and dependency on you, increase consultation opportunities, and help you keep an objective state of mind when making clinical decisions. In the current context, however, Laura may experience this suggestion as a rejection and resist it. It will probably take several discussions before she sees it as in her interest. Of course, this option presupposes that your patient can afford the added costs and that you have an available colleague.)

C. Explore her apparent dependency on you. [1] (Without shaming her, note that her panic about your absence is quite extraordinary. Educate her about interpersonal hypersensitivity, rejection sensitivity, and the basic attachment dilemmas in BPD. Then problem-solve about its management.)

D. Discuss your dilemma about hospitalization—that is, that it makes her safe but may become (or already has become) regressive and life-interfering. Note that "our failure" (thereby including yourself as part of the problem) to have a constructive conversation about this in your office reflects the fragility of this treatment. [1] (It is important to discuss the way in which the suicidal threats have an interpersonal impact on the treatment and treatment relationship.)

E. Be concerned about possible liability and seek forensic advice. [3] (This is overreactive. There is no indication of liability or legal concerns at this point. Such unwarranted fearfulness reflects failures of empathy and of wise assessment of risk. Consultation with other clinicians about one's own clinical judgment might be useful—certainly more useful than forensic advice.)

F. Suggest that she tell her family about what happened. [2] (This is generally a good idea. It is ideal to have families involved in the treatment for offspring with BPD. When safety issues are at hand, families benefit from having some education and can offer useful sources of support. However, Laura is 25 years old and has lived away from home for 7 years. Eventually, Laura disclosed more about her still emotionally [and financially] fraught relationship with her family. That lent itself to involving them.)

Case 5, Lawrence: Long-Term Therapy

Illustrating Chapters 2, 4, 6, and 7

This case involves an outpatient whose investment in treatment is sometimes in conflict with his preoccupation with relationships and with his habit of avoiding painful topics. It provides an example of long-term treatment wherein GPM's case management model evolves into a psychotherapy. Readers should note that the clinician doesn't always respond in the optimal ways. This illustrates that everyone makes mistakes, but their consequences are rarely very harmful. The report is divided into three parts. First, "Getting Started" illustrates issues with alliance building, self-disclosure, and evaluating progress. Second, "Settling In" issues include helping with school and romantic functioning—and the patient's tendency to avoid painful subjects. The third part, "Changes," sees the issues become more intrapsychic and explicitly includes the patient's relationship to the treater.

Part 1: Getting Started (the First 6 Months)
Illustrating Chapters 2, 4, and 6

Case Vignette: Getting Started

Lawrence, a 22-year-old single Asian second-year art school student, was referred to you after being discharged from a surgical ward where he had been hospitalized for a complex fracture of his wrist. The fracture occurred after he stepped off a stage while disrobed and intoxicated. During the hospitalization, his long-standing history of marijuana dependency and his recent history of increasing depression, insomnia, and passive suicidal ideation were noted. A psychiatric consultation was requested. The consultation showed an additional history of self-damaging behaviors (cutting and skin picking), adolescent cocaine abuse, uncontrolled anger, and terrifying nightmares. [**Decision Point 1**] He was given the diagnosis of BPD. His geographically distant parents were informed, and after the referral to you as an experienced BPD treater was made, they came to Boston.

Lawrence was a very thin, modestly unkempt, intense young man with a face scarred from recent picking. He appeared vigilant, clearly intelligent, and desperate for help. Lawrence said that he had diagnosed himself with BPD at age 14 and had always resented being misdiagnosed as bipolar, a diagnosis that had led to numerous failed medication trials. In his view, more injurious was that his parents had stopped listening to him and used the bipolar diagnosis as an explanation for all his subsequent problems. His parents too now embraced the new diagnosis and begged you, as an "expert," to "take him on." Lawrence too said that he thought that you could help him. You liked him, but being considered an "expert" made you apprehensive: apprehensive about initiating treatment during a crisis when expectations seemed unrealistically high—given his having failed many years of prior treatments and given your own record of inconsistent success. [**Decision Point 2**]

At Lawrence's request, you agreed to meet twice weekly. He asked whether you would stick with him if he got in trouble. You said that you would continue as long as you both felt it was helpful. You also told him that you both would need to pay attention to whether the therapy proved helpful. You encouraged him to write an autobiography and, because of his problems concentrating and sleeping, initiated arrangements for neuropsychiatric testing. He agreed with all these plans. Note that, without discussion, you quietly inherited the task of prescribing Prozac because it was prescribed long distance by a psychiatrist Lawrence had stopped seeing a year or so previously. [**Decision Point 3**]

He was silent to begin sessions, saying that he "had trouble knowing what to talk about." [**Decision Point 4**] You responded with questions about his school situation and family relationships. He also talked about his long-standing habits of truancy and risk-taking behaviors and his sense of badness since early childhood.

After the first three sessions, his attendance became inconsistent. Missed sessions usually were preceded by last-minute messages that he was ill (he often was), he needed to complete a school assignment, or the weather or other issues interfered with his commute. [**Decision Point 5**] On occasions when he missed without notifying you, you left messages querying about his welfare. Doing this via telephone messages proved futile (he never listened to them), so you began to e-mail "Where's Lawrence?" when you concluded that he wasn't coming. In response to his attendance problems, you reduced the frequency of appointments to once a week and rescheduled them for afternoons in deference to his dysfunctional sleep pattern. Attendance became somewhat more reliable. In time, when he knew he couldn't make it, some sessions were done by telephone.

Four months after starting, Lawrence unexpectedly announced that he was going skiing for spring break with classmates. [**Decision Point 6**] You advised him that he should prioritize his physical and mental health. He said that his friends were "counting" on him. He went and returned on crutches.

The content of sessions largely concerned classes and teachers he disliked, guilt and control struggles with friends (he "couldn't say no"), being chronically late and needing to cram on assignments, recurrent illnesses (related to poor sleep, diet, and exercise habits), and his upsetting communications with his long-term girlfriend. She was an unemployed college dropout who shared his marijuana habit and spent most of her time living in friends' apartments. "She's sort of a mooch," he said. You agreed.

His ongoing insomnia involved nightmares with vivid, horrifying images of torture. These seemed real to him, like flashbacks. He resisted exploring the links with past trauma. His ongoing abuse of marijuana was in part, he said, self-medication for his sleep problems. A trial of Ambien aggravated the nightmares. This led you to advise and arrange for a difficult-to-attain sleep consultation. He canceled it at the last minute, he said, because of examination pressure. He rescheduled it for the interval after school ended, but that appointment also eventually got canceled.

As school ended, Lawrence prepared to go home for the summer. Because his interactions with his family were often very angry, you questioned whether this was a good idea. He protested that summers at home were "wonderful"—including the prospect of being reunited with his girlfriend. As he prepared to go home, you asked for his assessment of his therapy. He noted that he had stopped drinking and that his suicidal ideas and depression were better. You agreed but told him that you often felt like a spectator who had failed to successfully involve him in the therapy. [**Decision Point 7**] When he asked why, you noted that sessions were largely about urgent current crises without much continuity or thematic depth. You noted that his attendance had been inconsistent, and he hadn't followed up on the sleep study, neuropsychiatric testing, or writing his autobiography. He looked hurt but then protested that "you are very important to me, and this therapy has been very valuable." [**Decision Point 8**]

Summary of Part 1

You have begun treatment with a patient who appeared to be desperate for help but who then proved difficult to engage. The first phase of treatment was concerned with recurrent crises and self-care. You are frustrated by failure to involve Lawrence more in treatment and to become someone he would lean on for help, but Lawrence has made some improvements in self-care and mood and seems to have a positive bond with you. It is worth noting that a less flexible treatment model (e.g., one that required regular appointments or one that precluded reaching out to the patient between sessions) might have either enlisted more involvement from Lawrence or precipitated Lawrence's departure.

Part 2: Settling In:
Approach/Avoidance Issues
(Junior and Senior Years in College)

Illustrating Chapters 2 and 6

Case Vignette: Settling In

Lawrence returned to school with enthusiasm and resumed seeing you once weekly—bicycling out to appointments. He looked strikingly better because he had gained weight, stopped face-picking, exercised regularly, and improved his grooming. He still had frequent nightmares and a thrice-daily marijuana habit. [**Decision Point 9**] You and he targeted better sleep hygiene, more self-assertiveness, and reduced marijuana use as goals. His sessions developed the theme of how failures to stand up for himself with friends, his girlfriend, and his parents were associated with poor self-esteem and unintentionally self-harmful behaviors.

On two occasions, Lawrence reached what you considered "breakthroughs" during which deep-seated feelings and memories emerged. After each event, however, Lawrence reverted to his old habits of missing sessions for illness, situational crises, weather, and so forth.

1. In October, he recalled traumatically being raped (sodomized while taking drugs) when he was 15 years old. He stumbled on this recall while describing a thoroughly dissolute drug and sex life, including multiple permanently scarring cuts, that took place defiantly under his parents' nose in early adolescence. This confirmed a posttraumatic stress disorder (PTSD) aspect to his psychology. [**Decision Point 10**] Your encouragement for him to resume talking about the event in subsequent sessions proved fruitless; "I just don't want to go there now."

2. While home in December, he discovered that his girlfriend was exchanging sexually explicit and flirtatious text messages with another man. This triggered disturbing memories of having observed his mother's infidelities when he was age 7. It also prompted him to consider leaving the "two-timing mooch" girlfriend—triggering fears of aloneness he considered intolerable: "I just can't deal with that right now."

During that Christmas break, he confronted his father about "finding excuses to be away" whenever he came home—acknowledging his hope for more of his father's attention. This was a big step. He felt reassured that his father "had actually listened to what I had to say." You applauded him for speaking up.

As winter moved to spring, you again inquired about his long-overdue autobiography. You had intermittently encouraged him to do this since the therapy had begun, but he repeatedly replied that he had started, had made progress, would bring it in, wasn't quite ready, needed more time, etc. [**Decision Point 11**] This time you volunteered to help him write it. He didn't object to or seem shamed by your assistance. As it progressed, you found it helpful to have a written ordering of his life events.

In April, after being invited and vetted and then having undergone extended screening for a prized award at his school, he was then rejected. He was initially rageful and self-pitying but eventually considered how rivalries and misinformation may have contributed to his having been rejected. This perspective taking was helped by having started a new romance. Feeling guilty about this, he broke off his relationship with the "two-timing mooch" back home. The new girlfriend was a somewhat quiet fellow student whose strong work ethic, intellectual ambitions, and quieter drug-free lifestyle contrasted with his prior relationship. You commented that this was a positive step but told him that having a period with no girlfriend would be helpful to his self-confidence and to shaping less needy partnerships. He completed the school year having completed his papers and examinations on schedule and having significantly elevated his grade point average. You questioned whether not going home for the summer would be a valuable separation from his family and would offer an opportunity to explore issues of his past, notably trauma, he had avoided. [**Decision Point 12**] He appeared to consider this but concluded that he really wanted to "get away."

It was a relatively peaceful summer for Lawrence. He maintained intermittent contact with you—usually prompted by rageful reactions. Notably, he was able to spend more "quality time" with his parents (especially his father). When Lawrence returned to his senior year of school and to therapy, he discussed how his parents had always perceived him as burdensome and that his girlfriend's and friends' loyalties to him were charitable. In fact, his mother had questioned his judgment for leaving his prior girlfriend "because she took care of you." Lawrence began to understand that his mother had, herself, compromised her self-esteem to stay in her marriage "to be taken care of." At one point in these discussions, you interrupted Lawrence's recurrent refrain about being lucky to have such a wonderful family, saying "No, I don't think that's true." "Well, it is much better than most." "No, I don't think you really think so; you have what I consider a dysfunctional family." "Still, I'm grateful." "No," you said, "I think you only think you should be." He seemed surprised by this interpretation but more thoughtful than upset. This exchange reflected your confidence that the patient could accept your challenge of his idealized perception of his family without turning on you—a real test of the strength of his alliance.

As Thanksgiving approached, Lawrence planned to stay with his girlfriend but then changed his mind "because my parents guilt-tripped me." When his girlfriend became angry at what she perceived to be his inability to stand up to them and his disregard for her plans, Lawrence got loudly and publicly angry at her, and she walked away. He then called you for support. Despite your having encouraged such calls, this was the first time he had called. Unfortunately, you were expected elsewhere. [**Decision Point 13**] He subsequently recalled knowledge of his mother's infidelities and had frightening flashbacks of possible childhood sexual trauma. As in the past, he then missed sessions for several weeks despite your "Where's Lawrence" e-mails. When he returned, as in the past, the memories and flashbacks were buried.

During his remaining semester, his life was relatively stable and his academic performance continued to improve. Yet as graduation approached, he had no plans for what he would do with his life. He thought that he would return home and "hang around." He was reluctant to stay in New York "just to do therapy," but he wanted to stay in touch with you ("the best therapist I've ever seen"). His parents met with you at graduation, and while grateful for his improvement, they privately expressed concerns about his returning home ("he gets so angry at us") and having no vocational plan. [**Decision Point 14**] After becoming visibly agitated ("hurt," "scared") when you raised the question of finding a therapist near home, Lawrence reiterated his appreciation for you. He returned home with his parents promising that he would either return or be in touch by telephone. Because his girlfriend was attending summer school, it seemed likely he might actually return.

Summary of Part 2

In this phase of treatment, Lawrence continued the work that he had begun in the first year; he has developed more behavioral controls, healthier relationships, and more investment in his education, and he has established a more stable alliance with you. He has flirted with real self-exploration and has been able to accept some uncomfortable insights, such as the reality about his dysfunctional family. Nevertheless, he continues to have nightmares, depend on marijuana, lose his temper, and be unable to integrate his highly disturbing memories or his past traumas into a coherent life narrative. Again, he runs from the opportunity to examine persisting identity and self-control issues and goes home instead. From a GPM perspective, this is okay—you don't want to push the ideal of personal awareness at the expense of adequate functioning. At the same time, you think he's still too handicapped to attain the life goals of fulfilling work and a secure partnership.

Part 3: Changes (The Last 9 Months)
Illustrating Chapters 2 and 7

Case Vignette: Changes

Three weeks later, Lawrence left a message that he needed to talk to you. When you spoke, he reported that he had discovered that his girlfriend was text messaging a guy, and he had then "gone ballistic"; he had actually hit her and then begged her to forgive him. In discussing this, he alternated between expressions of anger at her "betrayal," self-condemnation that he had "asked for this," shame at his hitting her, and fears of losing her. He said that his parents had "blamed me as usual for screwing up the relationship." He became enraged with them.

He seemed responsive to your expression of concern and quickly calmed down as he spoke. You set up a telephone session for the next day. During that session, he said: "I know I've been walking on eggshells. I get too angry, and I can't control it. I'm too dependent on my girlfriend and even on my parents." He said that your suggestion that he come back for more intensive treatment "probably made sense." You felt encouraged by his self-awareness and his apparent readiness to invest more in treatment.

Lawrence returned to treatment and to cohabiting with his girlfriend. You discussed how to intensify his treatment. [**Decision Point 15**] He said that he wanted to intensify his sessions with you, but he agreed to a consultation with a DBT specialist and to joining a group therapy. You arranged the consultation, helped him get started in group therapy (self-assessment), and told him that you would be glad to meet more often, but this should await the consultant's advice. He met with the consultant, who was impressed by his significant improvement and his strong attachment to you but concluded that his PTSD symptoms needed attention before he could make use of DBT. [**Decision Point 16**]

The consultant told Lawrence that he should enter an exposure therapy to work on past trauma. When Lawrence heard this, he became very frightened and angry. He protested to you that he hadn't returned for this, he didn't want to change treaters, and he didn't want to go into a hospital. You explained that he didn't have to do it, that you didn't want to stop being his therapist, and that you wouldn't want him to undertake such a treatment if it would mean hospitalization. That evening he called, very distraught, to say that he was terrified by flashbacks of his rape and couldn't control his crying. [**Decision Point 17**] You encouraged him to come in to see you the next day (Saturday), to which he said thanks and that he'd call you if he thought he needed to. He called the next day to report that he had spent most of the night recalling with great fear and shame details of his rape experience, that his girlfriend had held him and comforted him, and that he was exhausted and thought he'd be better off sleeping than coming in.

In subsequent weeks, he began seeing you three times a week and was early for appointments. He recalled the details of his rape with shame and eventually anger in sessions with you. Soon thereafter, he did this with great effect in the group he had become involved with. His sleep improved, and he began to have nonnightmare dreams that he wanted to "analyze." He also began to write a more detailed autobiography, completed psychopharmacology and dermatology consultations, and wrote self-disclosing but humorous "fiction" about his experiences in acting classes. He returned to school, taking classes in writing and journalism. He also worked part time at a shelter for battered women. He gradually became far less reactive to his father—seeing him less as distant and cruel and more as isolated and handicapped. He also began to experiment with going places and socializing without having his girlfriend accompany him. She objected, but he did it anyway. When one of his "fictional" stories was accepted for publication, he concluded that he would study journalism.

He was accepted into a highly rated school of journalism and then made plans to relocate. [**Decision Point 18**] Although his girlfriend objected, he expressed hopes that she would come with him, but he remained firm about his plans. You smiled and felt proud of him when he told you that he did this.

It was now more than 3.5 years since Lawrence first came to your office. As he prepared to leave, you asked him how he would characterize his relationship with you. He seemed surprised by the question, thought for a bit, and then said: "I think you're the first person in my life who I've been able to trust.... You know I really miss you when I'm away." You replied, "That's nice. [pause] Do you wonder whether I miss you?" "No, I never think much about that." He sighed. "I know you have always noticed when I missed sessions or a phone call, and I know you've often worried about me." You asked, "Will you want to see someone after you get settled in school?" He looked stricken, was quiet, and then said, "I'm not sure. I think I'd like to stay in touch with you if that's OK?" You said, "that's fine." You were aware of having tears in your eyes. [**Decision Point 19**]

Summary of Part 3

Lawrence made dramatic progress during this stage of his treatment. It is difficult to know whether his working through of his trauma was an inevitable extension of the strong alliance he had developed with his treater or was precipitated by the consultant's suggestion of its priority—and the threat of seeing a new therapist. The disclosure of the trauma and the involvement with a group were themselves corrective processes that involved more trust and closeness—and taking better care of himself. Then life took over.

This long-term treatment ends, as is common, by life's opportunities and responsibilities becoming a priority. Lawrence remembers his therapist's persistent reaching out to him during his missed appointments. He feels ready to move on and become independent even from his girlfriend. The therapist will surely miss him, and Lawrence is stronger for having internalized that.

Decision Points: Alternative Responses

(1 = will be helpful, 2 = possibly helpful, continuing reservations, 3 = not helpful—or even harmful)
See next subsection for discussion.

Part 1: Decision Points 1–8

1. Given this admittedly incomplete information, what diagnostic disorders would you consider likely and what priority would you give them?

Diagnosis	Likelihood	Priority
	(1 = yes, 2 = possible, 3 = no)	(1 = high, 2 = medium, 3 = low)
Borderline personality disorder	—	—
Major depressive disorder	—	—
Bipolar I disorder	—	—
Bipolar II disorder	—	—
Substance use disorder	—	—
Posttraumatic stress disorder	—	—
Sleep disorder	—	—
Antisocial personality disorder	—	—
Obsessive-compulsive personality disorder	—	—

2. Before agreeing to treat Lawrence, you should

   A. First attain a good history, including past records. ___
   B. Consider your initial reactions to Lawrence. ___
   C. Spend a few sessions getting to know the patient. ___

D. Inquire about current suicidal plans and the seriousness of past suicide attempts, and develop a safety plan. ___

E. Establish agreed-on goals. ___

3. Assuming responsibility for Lawrence's medication management

   A. Should be undertaken only after a careful review of past medication trials. ___

   B. Requires knowledge about the role of the various classes of medications in treating BPD. ___

   C. Requires knowledge about the adjunctive role and expectable benefits of medications. ___

   D. Is a task that should be kept separate from psychotherapy. ___

4. When Lawrence protests that he doesn't know what to talk about, you should

   A. Appreciate that many borderline patients have neurocognitive deficits that make it impossible for them to initiate conversation. ___

   B. Initiate discussions about issues you know are germane to his problems. ___

   C. Interpret the patient's "inability" as a defensive effort to avoid talking about his problems. ___

   D. Recruit Lawrence into seeing his silence as a problem to be solved and see whether discrete aspects of it can be targeted as goals for change. ___

5. In response to Lawrence's inconsistent attendance and his situational explanations, you should

   A. Tell Lawrence that his absences are making it hard for his therapy to be helpful. ___

   B. Express sympathy for his situational problems and say that you'll see him next time. ___

   C. Consider changing the schedule or frequency of appointments. ___

   D. Express concern about his situational problems and ask whether you could help him address them more effectively. ___

   E. Charge for the missed appointments. ___

   F. Call after waiting a respectable 15–20 minutes and request that he get in touch by telephone. ___

   G. Do nothing, and address it as a problem in the next session. ___

6. How should you respond to an unanticipated break in treatment?

   A. Ask him to consider his plan carefully given his desperate status a few months ago and his frequently missed appointments. ___
   B. Tell him that his absence will undermine the progress he might expect from his treatment. ___
   C. Don't make a big deal of it, but encourage him to keep in touch. ___
   D. Ask him to help you reconcile this departure with the seemingly desperate need for therapy that was evident when he started. ___

7. Telling Lawrence your concerns about his therapy's progress

   A. Is unnecessary and potentially destructive to the alliance. ___
   B. Reflects a legitimate concern that he has not made the expectable improvements.
   C. Is a valuable exercise. ___

8. How do you understand and respond to Lawrence's protestations of valuing therapy?

   A. You think he feels guilty and wants to placate you because he perceives that you are angry about his absences, failed homework, and impending departure. You ask whether he worries that you're angry. ___
   B. You think that what he said is probably true; that is, you have been more valuable as an "anchor to the wind" than you've realized. You signal your acceptance of his statement by nodding. ___
   C. You find this hard to understand, and you ask him to help you understand more about it. ___

Part 2: Decision Points 9–14

9. Lawrence's long-standing and unimproved marijuana habit (with only occasional attention during his prior 6 months in the treatment) calls for you to

   A. Remain concerned but wait until the patient identifies it as a priority he wants to work on. ___
   B. Encourage him to prioritize this issue. ___
   C. Make a point of giving more attention to this issue—by encouraging him to keep a diary and by bringing it up for review in sessions. ___
   D. Explore the benefits and drawbacks of his marijuana habit. ___

10. After Lawrence discloses a vivid account of past trauma, confirming prior suspicions of PTSD, his treater should

    A. Validate how horrible it was. ____

    B. Recognize that this important disclosure opens the door for corrective "working through" and encourage him to say more. ____

    C. Adopt a less exploratory and more supportive stance. ____

    D. Become psychoeducational about the role that trauma has in his insomnia/nightmares and problems with anger. ____

11. The failed autobiography homework: whether and how to respond:

    A. Stress how important the homework is for you to be able to make sense of his life. ____

    B. Give it up; if or when he wants to do this, he will. ____

    C. Volunteer to help him. ____

12. Should the therapist have impressed on Lawrence the need for integration of past trauma and suggested an intensified summer program?

    A. Yes. Without such integration, he faces an impaired career and impaired capability as a husband or father. ____

    B. No. He is not ready to take on such integration, and the effort required could further disrupt the natural maturational and developmental processes that are under way. ____

    C. Integration of his trauma should be encouraged with appropriate reservations about whether this is the best time to undertake this and about your ability to forecast how much it would affect his life.

____

13. When Lawrence calls in distress when you were about to leave for a family event, you should

    A. Listen briefly, and tell him you regrettably cannot talk now, but you will look forward to discussing this in your next session. ____

    B. Listen patiently as he airs out his problems. ____

    C. Let him know that you're glad he called. ____

14. In response to Lawrence's plan to return home and retain you on an as-needed basis, you

A. Conclude that we've done a good piece of work; it's okay to accept his plan. ___

B. Conclude that he remains ambivalent about staying involved in therapy and ask him to discuss this. ___

C. Invite Lawrence to consider whether he might do better with a different approach. ___

Part 3: Decision Points 15–19

15. In discussing how to intensify Lawrence's treatment, you

   A. Suggest that he convert to a BPD-specific treatment (e.g., DBT, Mentalization-Based Treatment [MBT], or transference-focused psychotherapy [TFP]). ___

   B. Encourage him to learn about BPD's evidence-based treatments and decide what he wants. ___

   C. Discuss available options and help him evaluate their potential value. ___

   D. Emphasize the value of adding a group therapy. ___

16. As the consultant who has reached these conclusions, you should

   A. Be frank with Lawrence about your impressions. ___

   B. Tell Lawrence that you will want to think more about your impressions and discuss them with his therapist before reaching any conclusions. ___

   C. Tell Lawrence some impressions and retain others. ___

17. In response to the resurgence of memories of his traumatic rape, you should

   A. Encourage him to go to an emergency department if he feels overwhelmed. ___

   B. Ask how you can be helpful. ___

   C. Note that, however unintentionally, he's begun to face the issues that he's been avoiding. ___

   D. Encourage him to do counting exercises, exercise, reading, or whatever might distract him. ___

   E. Inquire about his safety. ___

   F. Inquire about whether his girlfriend or others are available to give him support. ___

18. In response to Lawrence's intention to relocate, you should

  A. Inquire about the effect of leaving therapy. ___
  B. Suggest that he should first integrate his recent changes and establish their resilience before leaving. ___
  C. Applaud his dramatic improvement, and let him know you have confidence in his success. ___

19. How do you understand the relationship between Lawrence and his treater?

  A. The initial pursuit of him for missed appointments was needed. ___
  B. His resistance to seeing a new therapist reflects his inability to terminate with his therapist. ___
  C. The tearfulness of the therapist should have been suppressed. ___
  D. The treater has served the role of a surrogate parent. ___

Discussion

Part 1: Decision Points 1–8

1. Given this admittedly incomplete information, what diagnostic disorders would you consider likely and what priority would you give them ?

   (see "Comorbidities" in Chapter 6)

Diagnosis	Likelihood	Priority	Comments
	(1 = yes, 2 = possible, 3 = no)	(1 = high, 2 = medium, 3 = low)	
Borderline personality disorder	1	1	Anger, self-harm, help-seeking
Major depressive disorder	2	2	
Bipolar I disorder	3	3	No evidence of mania, elation
Bipolar II disorder	2	3	

Diagnosis	Likelihood	Priority	Comments
Substance use disorder	1	2	Becomes primary if causing ongoing dysfunction
Posttraumatic stress disorder (PTSD)	2	2	Nightmares, vigilance are suggestive
Sleep disorder	2	2	? Related to PTSD or situation
Antisocial personality disorder	3	3	
Obsessive-compulsive personality disorder	2	3	Too impulsive

2. Before agreeing to treat Lawrence, you should
   (see Chapter 4)

   A. First attain a good history, including past records. [2] (Getting a history and past records are desirable but time-consuming and sometimes unfeasible—as perhaps with this posthospital referral.)
   B. Consider your initial reactions to Lawrence. [1] (The relationship is real and professional. If you dislike or feel too anxious about a patient, it is wise to proceed with caution.)
   C. Spend a few sessions getting to know the patient. [2] (This is a good idea but often complicated by the urgency of a referring service [e.g., an inpatient setting] and by Lawrence's probable sensitivity to rejection after declaring his wish to work with you.)
   D. Inquire about current suicidal plans and the seriousness of past suicide attempts, and develop a safety plan. [3] (There is no reason to assume Lawrence is actively suicidal. In the absence of active suicidality, your emphasis on this issue is too reactive; it might unfortunately tilt your role toward safety management.)
   E. Establish agreed-on goals. [2] (This is a good idea but not a prerequisite to starting treatment. Setting goals encourages accountability, but establishing them can be a goal in its own right.)

3. Assuming responsibility for Lawrence's medication management

   (see "General Principles" and "Selecting Medications" in Chapter 6 and "Rationale" and "Selecting Another Modality" in Chapter 7)

   A. Should be undertaken only after a careful review of past medication trials. [3] (In principle, this is generally good, but with a borderline patient with a relatively simple task of managing a simple regimen, such a review would both distract from more important issues and could convey a misleading emphasis. Remember to be pragmatic: awaiting records can delay treatment and cause unnecessary complications.)
   B. Requires knowledge about the role of the various classes of medications in treating BPD. [2] (Such knowledge is useful, but it is important only if the patient has side effects or you are either consulting or needing to change medication.)
   C. Requires knowledge about the adjunctive role and expectable benefits of medications. [1] (Yes, giving them a primary role or encouraging strong benefits is almost always harmful. A cautious empirical approach is always desirable.)
   D. Is a task that should be kept separate from psychotherapy. [3] (These modalities are often easily combined. Lawrence's medication regimen is not complicated and is not a subject of immediate concern to him.)

4. When Lawrence protests that he doesn't know what to talk about, you should

   (see "Basic Therapeutic Approach" in Chapter 2; specific issue not covered in text)

   A. Appreciate that many borderline patients have neurocognitive deficits that make it impossible for them to initiate conversation. [3] (They may occasionally have neurocognitive problems, but even then it rarely explains this common issue. This is almost always an issue of intrapsychic and interpersonal anxiety. Suggesting and pursuing a neurocognitive explanation not only is not helpful but also moves the patient into a role as a passive victim of his or her disorder rather than someone who can and should try to develop competence.)
   B. Initiate discussions about issues you know are germane to his problems. [1] (Be active. This is especially necessary in the early parts of therapies when the borderline patient's problem with

speaking probably reflects anxiety about the situation and you. Of course, this approach doesn't directly address or resolve Lawrence's reason for not talking.)

C. Interpret the patient's "inability" as a defensive effort to avoid talking about his problems. [3] (This might be correct but will likely make the patient more defensive. "Interpretations" can be given indirectly; in this case, by inquiring about whether Lawrence feels anxious about the therapy—or about you. This would be more facilitative. This actively involves the patient in his or her own self-examination. If Lawrence acknowledges such anxieties, offer him an education about therapy and try to reassure him.)

D. Recruit Lawrence into seeing his silence as a problem to be solved and see whether discrete aspects of it can be targeted as goals for change. [2] (This approach usefully sees his problem initiating sessions as being within himself and that he can work on it, but it overlooks the problem's immediate situational and interpersonal origins. Moreover, it seems unlikely that Lawrence could undertake this collaboration at this point. This approach would be more promising if Lawrence described similar problems in many social situations. Otherwise, it may be time-consuming and still not yield communications about more pressing issues.)

5. In response to Lawrence's inconsistent attendance and his situational explanations, you should

(see "Basic Therapeutic Approach" in Chapter 2; specific problem not covered in text)

A. Tell Lawrence that his absences are making it hard for his therapy to be helpful. [2] (This is a good message, but it might evoke his shame [he's bad] or anger [you're critical]. Why he is missing appointments needs to be addressed first. Although you might be helpful to him even through missed appointments, it is useful for you both to stay aware that being helpful determines whether the therapy will persist.)

B. Express sympathy for his situational problems and say that you'll see him next time. [3] (This is too passive—the missed appointments are a problem that needs to be addressed as such. When situational explanations are repeated, it is unlikely to be "situational.")

C. Consider changing the schedule or frequency of appointments. [2] (It is generally wise to decrease the frequency when a patient doesn't attend, but understanding the reasons for missing remains a priority. To sustain your holding function, you want to convey that you don't agree with your patient's avoidance of issues that might better be discussed. With respect to schedule changes, try to accommodate patients unless it is inconvenient for you, and if it is, then say so.)

D. Express concern about his situational problems and ask whether you could help him address them more effectively. [1] (This response takes the missed sessions seriously and shows a real interest in his life outside of sessions. How you raise the sensitive issue of managing the situations "more effectively" is critical. If becoming more effective is posed as your expectation, some patients will feel criticized and get more defensive. If it is posed as an invitation to problem solve ["Might I help you consider ways to..."], it usually will be rewarded.)

E. Charge for the missed appointments. [2] (This is a good idea insofar as it holds the patient responsible and your time as valuable, but patients should be prepared for this—including the fact that insurance will not usually cover it.)

F. Call after waiting a respectable 15–20 minutes, and do the rest of the session by telephone. [3] (This risks reinforcing missed appointments and implies too little accountability.)

G. Do nothing, and address it as a problem in the next session. [1] (Generally, this is the best strategy. It's the patient's loss, isn't it?)

6. How should you respond to an unanticipated break in treatment?

(see "Basic Therapeutic Approach" in Chapter 2; specific issue not covered in text)

A. Ask him to consider his plan carefully given his desperate status a few months ago and his frequently missed appointments. [1] (This is worth discussing and does convey your concern and involvement.

B. Tell him that his absence will undermine the progress he might expect from his treatment. [3] (This response is likely to be experienced as controlling. It contrasts with Good Psychiatric Management's focus on getting a life and could encourage dependency on treatment.)

C. Don't make a big deal of it. [2] (Failure to express concern about his absence will be experienced as not caring. Too much concern is inconsistent with the "get a life" message.)

D. Ask him to help you reconcile this departure with the seemingly desperate need for therapy that was evident when he started. [2] (This invites him to think about his decision, but it also conveys your disapproval—for better or worse.)

7. Telling Lawrence your concerns about his therapy's progress

(see "Basic Therapeutic Approach" and "How Change Occurs" in Chapter 2 and "Setting the Framework" in Chapter 4)

A. Is unnecessary and potentially destructive to the alliance. [3] (In therapy with borderline patients, continuation should be contingent on such ongoing evaluation of progress—as was planned with Lawrence from the start. It may hurt a self-object form of relatedness, but it helps establish and sustain a collaborative working alliance.)

B. Reflects a legitimate concern that he has not made the expectable improvements. [2] (As is expectable, his acute symptoms, level of distress, and suicidal/self-harm acts have decreased. Moreover, you like and feel liked by the patient. But Lawrence's investment and involvement in the tasks are unclear—ambivalent at best. He shows little evidence of thinking about prior discussions or lessons learned. So, raising the question of the therapy's value is by these standards optional.)

C. Is a valuable exercise. [1] (Expectations of positive change were part of the initial discussions. It is easy for therapies that are mutually satisfactory to overlook whether change is occurring. Conjoint examination of progress is good.)

8. How do you understand and respond to Lawrence's protestations of valuing therapy?

(see "Basic Therapeutic Approach" and "How Change Occurs" in Chapter 2; specific issue not covered in text)

A. You think he feels guilty and wants to placate you because he perceives that you are angry about his absences, failed homework, and impending departure. You ask whether he worries that you're angry. [2] (This explanation is a reasonable possibility, and the interpretation—by way of a question—is good. Even if it is correct, however, he might not be able to own such worries. Also, there might be other explanations.)

B. You think that what he said is probably true; that is, you have been more valuable as an "anchor to the wind" than you've realized. You signal your acceptance of his statement by nodding. [2] (This is a reasonable possibility, and the response follows from it. This is consistent with the GPM model of using you as a transitional object: he knew he could call you as-needed; you were silently essential and trustworthy—modeling thoughtfulness and self-controls for him to introject. It should not, however, erase other possible explanations, such as response A for this discussion.)

C. You find this hard to understand, and you ask him to help you understand more about it. [1] (This shows your interest and doesn't convey either skepticism or acceptance.)

Part 2: Decision Points 9–14

9. Lawrence's long-standing and unimproved marijuana habit (with only occasional attention during his prior 6 months in the treatment) calls for you to

(see "Basic Therapeutic Approach" in Chapter 2; specific problem not addressed in text)

A. Remain concerned but wait until the patient identifies it as a priority he wants to work on. [2] (As long as it is not interfering with his functioning [to your knowledge] and he knows that his habit concerns you, this forbearance is probably wise. Marijuana may have stabilizing functions he's not ready to give up.)

B. Encourage him to prioritize this issue. [3] (It isn't clear that this issue should be his first priority, or that he wants to change his habit, or that it is seriously handicapping his functioning.)

C. Make a point of giving more attention to this issue—by encouraging him to keep a diary and by bringing it up for review in sessions. [2] (This does underscore your concern and might make his marijuana habit more dystonic to him. But, in the absence of its interfering with his life and given his history of failing to follow up on prior homework or on consultations that you've encouraged, this focus seems unlikely to be effective.)

D. Explore the benefits and drawbacks of his marijuana habit [1] (This so-called motivational interviewing technique opens up the topic and will make it clear whether to give this issue more attention. It is also in keeping with the GPM principle of keeping the patient an active participant in treatment.)

10. After Lawrence discloses a vivid account of past trauma, confirming prior suspicions of PTSD, his treater should

(see "How Change Occurs" in Chapter 2 and "Comorbidities" in Chapter 6)

A. Validate how horrible it was. [1] (Yes, in general such responses are always helpful for patients to own their experiences and feel understood.)

B. Recognize that this important disclosure opens the door for corrective "working through" and encourage him to say more. [2] (Working through is possible but usually will not occur until the patient's alliance is firm and his or her outside life is stable; neither is the case with Lawrence.)

C. Adopt a less exploratory and more supportive stance. [3] (Insofar as the therapeutic stance has already been supportive, becoming more so might be patronizing or encourage a victim identification. Those effects unwittingly discourage "working through." Concerned curiosity should be sustained.)

D. Become psychoeducational about the role that trauma has in his insomnia/nightmares and problems with anger. [1] (This is a good idea—helping him see the possible benefits of later "working through.")

11. The failed autobiography homework: whether and how to respond

(see "Building an Alliance" and "Common Problems" in Chapter 4)

A. Stress how important the homework is for you to be able to make sense of his life. [3] (It is certainly understandable that a therapist can feel confused in the absence of knowing the patient's sequence of events and how they are related. But, as stated, this is for your sake. Have confidence that your inability to make sense of his life will get corrected if and as Lawrence can tolerate it.)

B. Give it up; if or when he wants to do this, he will. [2] (This is probably true, but it indicates that you actually don't place much value on it.)

C. Volunteer to help him. [2] (Doing this underscores your belief that a coherent personal narrative is important, but it runs counter to the issue of personal accountability. It is probably only worthwhile if the homework—in this case, Lawrence's history of major life events—is a task that you feel the patient can benefit from.)

12. Should the therapist have impressed on Lawrence the need for integration of past trauma and suggested an intensified summer program?

    (see "Basic Therapeutic Approach" in Chapter 2 and "Impending Self-Endangering Behaviors" in Chapter 5)

    A. Yes. Without such integration, he faces an impaired career and impaired capability as a husband or father. [3] (We can't be sure how damaging these traumas will remain. Moreover, we can't be sure that the desired integration would occur from a more intensive treatment. Life and maturation can be healing. Moreover, being very insistent on this issue could risk disrupting the improved relationship he has made with you.)
    B. No. He is not ready to take on such integration, and the effort required could further disrupt the natural maturational and developmental processes that are under way. [3] (You can't know whether he's ready. He's proceeding as a college student, but his life is still interrupted by crises and avoidance.)
    C. Integration of his trauma should be encouraged with appropriate reservations about whether this is the best time to undertake this and about your ability to forecast how much it would affect his life. [1] (Yes.)

13. When Lawrence calls in distress when you were about to leave for a family event, you should

    A. Listen briefly, and tell him you regrettably cannot talk now, but you will look forward to discussing this in your next session. [2] (A reasonable response that may, however, undermine what has been a significant step forward by Lawrence.)
    B. Listen patiently as he airs out his problems. [1] (This is basically the best approach for Lawrence, for whom asking for help has been difficult. Patient listening is a sound approach to most distressed first calls. Still, your conflicting agenda needs to be given due consideration.)
    C. Let him know that you're glad he called. [1] (By now, you know that there's no risk of this privilege being abused by this patient.)

14. In response to Lawrence's plan to return home and retain you on an as-needed basis, you

A. Conclude that we've done a good piece of work; it's okay to accept his plan. [3] (He's completed college and has a more stable romantic partner, but his continued problems with anger, unstable relationships, and past trauma greatly handicap his future. His avoidance needs to be challenged.)

B. Conclude that he remains ambivalent about staying involved in therapy and ask him to discuss this. [1] (Yes, it seems apparent that he needs but fears any commitments.)

C. Invite Lawrence to consider whether he might do better with a different approach. [1] (This is a good question. Raising it with Lawrence at this point would certainly be a good idea. He might indicate that you present problems that can't be solved [e.g., your gender, style]. It also might encourage him to voice objectives he otherwise wouldn't. Because raising this question might be experienced as your interest in withdrawing, it should be accompanied by a statement of your interest in continuing.)

Part 3: Decision Points 15–19

15. In discussing how to intensify Lawrence's treatment, you

A. Suggest that he convert to a BPD-specific treatment (e.g., DBT, Mentalization-Based Treatment [MBT], or Transference-Focused Psychotherapy [TFP]). [2] (This is rather precipitous after working together for more than 2 years, and, insofar as it involves a new individual therapist, this suggestion will invoke rejection anxieties. Still TFP, DBT, and MBT offer ways to enhance what you are offering, and he should be encouraged to consider them.)

B. Encourage him to learn about BPD's evidence-based treatments and decide what he wants. [3] (It isn't as if the evidence-based treatments are likely to be available. Moreover, the selection of any of them must consider your ability to collaborate with the specific practitioners and your judgment about their skills. Also, Lawrence's decision should be informed by what you recommend and why. DBT, for example, may be optimal for patients with a pattern of dangerous self-harm who feel comfortable with didactics, whereas TFP might be optimal for patients with stable employment who need to be challenged.)

C. Discuss available options and help him evaluate their potential value. [1] (The options are usually quite discrete and only occasionally will include evidence-based treatments provided by capable clinicians. Involving the patient in choosing is always a good idea.)

D. Emphasize the value of adding a group therapy. [1] (Yes, this is almost always the most cost-effective modality to add. The suggestion usually meets with resistance, so you need to urge it, explain its merits, and be persistent!)

16. As the consultant who has reached these conclusions, you should

A. Be frank with Lawrence about your impressions. [2] (Although this often is good procedure for patients who seek consultation, it is complicated here because this consultation came from a colleague [the primary therapist] who remains responsible for the patient's treatment and because the attachment to that therapist will make the recommendation to initiate a previously undiscussed form of therapy [i.e., expressive therapy] very destabilizing.)

B. Tell Lawrence that you will want to think more about your impressions and discuss them with his therapist before reaching any conclusions. [2] (This generally conservative approach will frustrate the patient and undermine the authority attributed to the consultant. Some conclusions are safely imparted [e.g., about the considerable improvement, about the wisdom of investing more in treatment, and that the relationship with the primary therapist has been valuable].)

C. Tell Lawrence some impressions and retain others. [1] (This follows from the previous discussion of A and B alternatives.)

17. In response to the resurgence of memories of his traumatic rape, you should

A. Encourage him to go to an emergency department if he feels overwhelmed. [3] (This response would aggravate his fears of hospitalization and be perceived as a sign of your inability or unwillingness to help with issues you've encouraged him to address.)

B. Ask how you can be helpful. [1] (This underscores his agency—requests that he be proactive on behalf of his own safety.)

C. Note that, however unintentionally, he's begun to face the issues that he's been avoiding. [1] (Yes, you don't want to cheerlead this, but you want to remind him of the potential progress.)

D. Encourage him to do counting exercises, exercise, reading, or whatever might distract him. [2] (This could be helpful, but it should be a secondary strategy. Lawrence has avoided recovery and integration of these memories, and the fact that he is committed to intensifying treatment means that this is a positive opportunity.)

E. Inquire about his safety. [3] (It is generally harmful to equate being upset with suicidality. Lawrence has made no indication of such risk.)

F. Inquire about whether his girlfriend or others are available to give him support. [1] (Yes, finding use of nontherapy support should be Lawrence's first strategy.)

18. In response to Lawrence's intention to relocate, you should

A. Inquire about the effect of leaving therapy. [1] (This is definitely important in both evaluating his readiness to leave and introducing the process of termination.)

B. Suggest that he should first integrate his recent changes and establish their resilience before leaving. [2] (It is a good question to raise, but to discourage his relocation because of this uncertainty runs counter to the "get a life" message.)

C. Applaud his dramatic improvement, and let him know you have confidence in his success. [3] (It is good to applaud his recent changes, but being confident about his proposed move will inhibit discussion of the obstacles he will encounter and exaggerate his sense of failing—and failing you—if he does not succeed.)

19. How do you understand the relationship between Lawrence and his treater?

A. The initial pursuit of him for missed appointments was needed. [2] (That Lawrence remembers and cites this establishes its importance to him. It remains possible that he would have become attached and gotten involved in therapy without this.)

B. His resistance to seeing a new therapist reflects his inability to terminate with his therapist. [3] (This response is too negative. It more likely testifies to realistic appreciation that his life change will consume most of his energies, that his current [past] therapist would be more helpful than anyone new, and that it will facilitate his moving on to know that such a resource remains available.)

C. The tearfulness of the therapist should have been suppressed. [3] (Although as a professional, one might feel self-conscious about this, for Lawrence the tears will only confirm that the relationship with his therapist has been real.)

D. The treater has served in the role of a surrogate parent. [2] (Certainly the therapist has served the stabilizing, guiding, and loving roles associated with being a good parent, and these have been corrective experiences. But the therapist has also been a hired professional whose wisdom and concern were paid for. This departs from a parental role.)

Case 6, Melanie: A Failed Split Treatment

Illustrating Chapter 7

A split treatment ends abruptly and shows instructive lessons about both patient and treater contributions, alliances, and the power and the limitations of idealized transferences.

Case Vignette

Melanie's dynamically oriented therapy with you (Dr. A) was productive, characterized by a growing attachment and dependency but also by persistent high-risk episodes of unsafe sex and driving under the influence. For your forthcoming 3-week vacation, you arranged coverage for Melanie by Dr. B. Dr. B was an experienced behaviorally oriented female colleague who had seen Melanie previously. In your absence, the therapy with Dr. B, focusing on skills, went well, and when you returned, it was agreed that Melanie should continue to see Dr. B for added support and more skills work. [**Decision Point 1**]

Soon after you resumed therapy, Melanie began to discuss incidents of cruel verbal abuse by her mother. You encouraged this, but in a session when you had asked for more details, she suddenly became frightened, then mute, shaking her head that she couldn't say more. You responded with sympathy and asked, "What just happened here?" She said that she thought you might tell her sister. Surprised, you asked, "What makes you think that I might do that?" She shook her head and said that she needed to leave. When she missed her next session, and didn't respond to your call, you informed Dr. B.

Melanie subsequently told Dr. B that she wouldn't go back to see you—citing again her suspicions about your intentions. [**Decision Point 2**] Dr. B neither validated nor expressed skepticism about Melanie's suspicions of you. She urged her to address her fears directly by talking with you. Melanie replied, "Maybe someday, but I don't feel safe going to see him now." When Dr. B repeated her suggestion, Melanie became angry. In the face of Melanie's angry resistance, Dr. B backed off and thereby implicitly (and silently) assumed the role of the primary therapist. [**Decision Point 3**]

A few weeks later, you called Dr. B to learn what was happening. Dr. B recounted what she called "Melanie's paranoid response" and her angry refusal to talk with you about it. You expressed surprise at Melanie's persistent suspicions and disappointment that what had seemed like a real step forward in Melanie's therapy had been so abruptly terminated. (Privately, you thought that Dr. B was colluding with the patient's avoidance by not protesting your integrity.) **[Decision Point 4]** You advised Dr. B that you still thought that Melanie's safety was better managed by a split treatment. You also encouraged Dr. B to get a consultation. Dr. B said that she felt comfortable seeing the patient alone, adding that she needed to establish a firmer alliance before getting a consultation.

Six months later, the patient was still attending therapy with Dr. B regularly and had joined a group run by her. She had not returned to see you or to the subject of her sexual abuse. Dr. B had made no contact with you. When you asked Dr. B about Melanie, Dr. B reported that she remained paranoid about you. What had happened? **[Decision Point 5]**

In retrospect, this split treatment failed for several reasons. First, when Dr. B was added, the contract was not clarified (i.e., about Dr. A's role as the primary clinician and about the open communications between the treaters). Second, Dr. B failed to challenge Melanie's inherently paranoid fears about Dr. A and failed to sustain the split treatment's structure by neither talking with Dr. A (with or without Melanie's presence) about her taking over his role nor seeking (with or without Melanie's permission) an outside consultant. The case illustrates how such a patient can play on clinicians' failures to establish and uphold a frame. Should the patient be faulted when such a failed split treatment occurs?

Decision Points: Alternative Responses

(1 = will be helpful, 2 = possibly helpful, continuing reservations, 3 = not helpful—or even harmful)

See next subsection for discussion.

1. The agreement to add Dr. B to Melanie's ongoing treatment

    A. Invites splitting. ___
    B. Is a poor combination of therapies. ___
    C. Requires a definition of roles, including who is the primary treater. ___
    D. Is inherently problematic because one therapist is psychodynamic and the other is behavioral. ___

2. When Melanie tells Dr. B that she distrusts you (Dr. A) and doesn't want to see you again, Dr. B should

    A. Ask the patient for permission to discuss the situation with you.

    ___

    B. Encourage Melanie to discuss her suspicions directly with you. ___

    C. Explore what prompted Melanie's conclusions about you. ___

    D. Tell her she might be right, but it's between her and Dr. A. ___

    E. Remain neutral—neither protect Dr. A nor validate the accusation. ___

3. When Melanie angrily refused to talk with you (Dr. A), Dr. B should

    A. Drop the subject, lest the patient become paranoid toward her. ___

    B. Tell Melanie that she is making a big mistake and she stands to learn a great deal by talking with you about this. ___

    C. Tell Melanie that she (Dr. B) could accept the change in treatment only after discussing this and obtaining agreement from you. ___

    D. Convey to Melanie that she (Dr. B) feels comfortable with this change, and resume her former role as primary therapist. ___

4. When Dr. B tells you that Melanie will not meet with you, you should

    A. Urge Dr. B to suspend their therapy until the patient has come to see you. ___

    B. Express concern about Melanie's safety risk with only one treater. Remind Dr. B that you encouraged her addition to the treatment because of your concerns about those safety risks. ___

    C. Suggest that Dr. B insist that they meet Melanie together. ___

    D. Wish Dr. B well. ___

    E. Tell Dr. B to defer any decision about assuming the role of primary therapist until after a consultation. ___

5. In retrospect, what could you say about the therapeutic relationship you had with Melanie at the time she dropped out (1=yes, 2=partly, 3=no)?

    A. A good working alliance had been established. ___

    B. You had established a good contractual alliance; i.e., you had agreed on roles and goals. ___

    C. Your alliance and her progress had been reliant on an idealized transference. ___

    D. You were "split" out of the treatment because of an unexplained transference reaction. ___

    E. Dr. B had inherited a similarly fragile idealized transference that was sustained by her willingness to avoid challenging Melanie. ___

Discussion

1. The agreement to add Dr. B to Melanie's ongoing treatment

    (see "Rationale" and "Selecting Another Modality" in Chapter 7)

    A. Invites splitting. [3] (No, most split treatments work well; it depends entirely on how well the split treatment is structured.)
    B. Is a poor combination of therapies. [2] (Both are individual therapists; hence their roles are likely to overlap, and the relative cost benefits of adding a second individual therapist compared with another modality are limited. In this case, however, these disadvantages are partly offset by distinctive therapy styles and by the patient's familiarity and comfort with Dr. B.)
    C. Requires a definition of roles, including who is the primary treater. [1] (Absolutely. Even among colleagues, it is useful to be clear about roles and communications.)
    D. Is inherently problematic because one therapist is psychodynamic and the other is behavioral. [3] (Different orientations can be complementary—it becomes problematic only when the clinicians do not understand and respect each other and what each is doing.)

2. When Melanie tells Dr. B that she distrusts you (Dr. A) and doesn't want to see you again, Dr. B should

    (see "Rationale" and "Common Problems" in Chapter 7)

    A. Ask the patient for permission to discuss the situation with you. [3] (Having such a discussion is a prerequisite expectation for split treatment. It should not be up to the patient's discretion.)
    B. Encourage Melanie to discuss her suspicions directly with you. [1] (Yes, this is basic, giving Melanie an active role in correcting her conflict and offering an opportunity for a corrective experience.)
    C. Explore what prompted Melanie's conclusions about you. [1] (This is definitely a good idea—with the hope that both you and the patient can evaluate whether the suspicion is warranted. You act like a consultant or marriage counselor.)
    D. Tell her she might be right, but it's between her and Dr. A. [3] (This indicates that Dr. B believes Melanie's suspicions are plausible. This response will make it less likely that the patient would talk to you [Dr. A].)

    E. Remain neutral—neither protect Dr. A nor validate the accusation. [1] (This is a good introductory stance, but assuming Dr. B doesn't believe Melanie's fears are realistic, this needs to be followed by response C and, if necessary, suggesting a conjoint meeting with her and Dr. A.)

3. When Melanie angrily refused to talk with you (Dr. A), Dr. B should

  (see "Common Problems" in Chapter 7)

    A. Drop the subject, lest the patient become paranoid toward her. [1] (The patient should be aware that you disapprove of her refusal to meet with you, but when her resistance got aggravated, it was best to back off.)

    B. Tell Melanie that she is making a big mistake—she stands to learn a great deal by talking with you about this. [1] (Therapists should be clear and explicit about supporting such a talk, explaining that it provides a valuable opportunity for patients to test their fears and assert themselves.)

    C. Tell Melanie that she (Dr. B) could accept the change in treatment only after discussing this and obtaining agreement from you. [1] (This conforms to the framework in which split treatments are established and actively counters any splits between treaters. It also is what the patient will probably expect. In that case, the failure to do this requires patients with BPD to split off such doubts to preserve a "goal" [idealized] treater.)

    D. Convey to Melanie that she (Dr. B) feels comfortable with this change, and resume her former role as primary therapist. [3] (Dr. B may feel that Melanie needs such reassurance, but it directly enacts the patient's split [A becomes "all bad"; B becomes "all good"]. It is easy to say Melanie caused this, but that conclusion would overlook the misinformed and highly significant contribution made by Dr. B.)

4. When Dr. B tells you that Melanie will not meet with you, you should

  (see "Common Problems" in Chapter 7)

    A. Urge Dr. B to suspend their therapy until the patient had come to see you. [2] (This upholds the agreement about your primary role but runs the real risk, if Melanie is truly paranoid about you, of leaving this risky patient with no treater.)

B. Express concern about Melanie's safety risk with only one treater. Remind Dr. B that you encouraged her addition to the treatment because of your concerns about those safety risks. [1] (This is a reasonable collegial admonishment.)

C. Suggest that Dr. B insist that they meet Melanie together. [1] (This is a good plan, affirming the structure of good split treatment.)

D. Wish Dr. B well. [3] (This would be deferring without protesting to a change you don't agree with.)

E. Tell Dr. B to defer any decision about assuming the role of primary therapist until after a consultation. [1] (This delays your official suspension without disrupting Melanie's ongoing therapy. The consultant should be someone both Dr. A and Dr. B can agree to.)

5. In retrospect, what could you say about the therapeutic relationship you had with Melanie at the time she dropped out (1 = yes, 2 = partly, 3 = no)?

(see Chapter 4 and Chapter 7)

A. A good working alliance had been established. [3] (This advanced form of alliance would have permitted the patient to stay in the office with you despite her distrust and consider it as a symptom to be examined. Her inability to do this, even when Dr. B encouraged her, testifies to how far she was from this form of alliance.)

B. You had established a good contractual alliance; i.e., you had agreed on roles and goals. [2] (The patient had been collaborating without contesting these issues. In retrospect, your role and responsibilities as her primary therapist had not been clarified either with the patient or with Dr. B.)

C. Your alliance and her progress had been reliant on an idealized transference. [1] (Yes, this aspect of the relationship had without a doubt motivated her to move into issues too readily. It was inherently fragile and was abruptly ended.)

D. You were "split" out of the treatment because of an unexplained transference reaction. [1] (Yes, this occurred, and neither you nor Dr. B has yet understood it. In retrospect, discussing mother's attacks may have triggered fears that Dr. A would do this; we don't know. Nor should we lose sight of the contributions to being "split out of the treatment" that derived from the unmade contract and by Dr. B's failing to stand by Dr. A.)

E. Dr. B had inherited a similarly fragile idealized transference that was sustained by her willingness to avoid challenging Melanie. [1]

(Yes, it is surprising that it has been sustained. Perhaps an unexamined gender issue also helped this.)

Case 7, Jill: Someone's BPD Here

Illustrating "Family Interventions" in Chapter 7

The chronically bitter alienation experienced within many families that have a member with BPD is both evoked by that offspring's angry hypersensitivity and provoked by reactive, inconsistent parenting. In this case, the treater finds a way to interrupt such a stalemate.

Case Vignette

Worried-looking middle-aged parents bring their 19-year-old daughter (Jill) to you for treatment. They listen quietly as Jill reluctantly describes her long history of self-injurious behavior, substance abuse, unsafe sex, and bulimia. Jill grows increasingly angry as she then builds the case that her parents were too preoccupied with themselves and with her mentally retarded younger sister to have given her the attention she needed. She calms somewhat when her father guiltily confesses to having lost his temper and having several times hit Jill when she was in grade school. But when her mother then describes violent fights with Jill, which have prompted her to call 911, Jill interrupts to say, "You caused the fights, Mom!" The parents look helplessly at each other and then turn to you. After a brief silence, they say how much they love Jill and promise that they will do whatever you advise, but "please, please take our daughter on. She needs you." The extreme tensions within the family are obvious, but you like Jill's animation and feel sympathetic to her parents' helplessness. You agree to see Jill weekly on a trial basis. You advise the parents to join a family support group and provide them with the contact information. As they leave, they express appreciation and ask, "May we call you if we have questions?" [**Decision Point 1**]

A few months pass. Jill's sessions are primarily concerned with a current situation (i.e., a boyfriend's loyalties and what she describes as her sister's attention-seeking dependency). She has generally resisted your efforts to say more about her relationship with her parents. When pushed, Jill reports that she can't eat meals with her mother because they "push each other's buttons." When you note that you haven't heard from her parents, Jill replies, "What did you expect? They're just happy I'm seeing you." She adds that they didn't join the family group and "that's fine by me." [**Decision Point 2**]

You tell Jill that her parents' failure to follow up on your advice concerns you. You say: "They should at least be educated about your disorder. Beyond that, I think their involvement would be helpful—your parents should become aware of how their responses can aggravate or ameliorate your problems." Jill agrees with this and agrees to your contacting them and inviting them to come in. But, she then insists, she will need to attend, and she needs to be informed in advance of what you plan to say to them. [**Decision Point 3**]

The family meeting is planned with Jill in attendance. The session began with her mother citing ongoing fights, then criticizing Jill for being disrespectful and for denying her role in starting these fights. Jill became enraged and said, "I don't have to listen to this same old bullshit." An escalating exchange ensues, and your efforts, assisted meekly by her father, fail to interrupt this. You ask Jill and her father to step outside into the waiting room. After they depart, her mother tearfully complains that "this is typical; I always walk on eggshells when she's around. I can't speak openly in front of her." She acknowledged how hurt she is by Jill's hostility but, when asked, failed to see her role in triggering Jill. You pointed out that this session had begun with her criticism of Jill for starting their fights. She failed to understand why Jill could have felt attacked, noting only that "Jill's the one who got angry!" You sympathize with how difficult it is to be attacked for failing as a mother. She welcomes this and begins to cry. You reiterate your prior recommendation that they join a parents' group, but now you add, with apprehension, that you recommend that she attain personal counseling "to learn not to take Jill's anger so personally." To your relief, she seems receptive. You give her several counselors' names to call.

In subsequent meetings with Jill, it was apparent that she felt validated by your recommending therapy for her mother. She recounted recurrent "verbal abuse" by her since childhood. At one point, she sadly concluded that maybe her mother had always disliked her. She felt discouraged about the prospect of her mother's changing, noting that her parents still hadn't followed up by joining the parents' group and that her mother hadn't contacted the therapists you had recommended. [**Decision Point 4**] You tell Jill that her mother becomes defensive when she is told that she's failed to be a good mother. You go on to tell Jill that one of your goals is to help her mother see things from Jill's perspective but that she, Jill, also needs to work on seeing herself from her mother's perspective.

In the months that followed, you sent mother and father the "Guidelines for Families" (see Appendix D) and then met with them to discuss them. Jill welcomed this. At that point, her parents began attending the parents' group, where her father soon became an enthusiastic leader. Mom and Jill gradually became less critical toward each other. Another 6 months later, mother suggested that she and Jill go out to a movie and dinner, leaving dad to care for the younger sister. Mother never reopened the question of therapy for herself.

Decision Points: Alternative Responses

(1 = will be helpful, 2 = possibly helpful, continuing reservations, 3 = not helpful—or even harmful)
See next subsection for discussion.

1. In response to the parents' inquiry about calling you, you respond

   A. That you'd like to talk with them but that you will have to get Jill's permission before you will be able to respond to their questions.

   ___

    B. That you would like to hear from them if they are concerned about Jill's safety or progress, or about the bills, but cannot discuss what goes on in sessions. ___

    C. That you try to keep families involved, so you make yourself available on an as-needed basis. ___

2. When you learn that Jill's parents didn't follow up on your advice, you should

    A. Do nothing. ___

    B. Recognize that her parents are enacting their daughter's primary complaint: they don't want to get involved with her problems. ___

    C. Tell Jill that you'd like to follow up on having her parents join a group, but ask whether she's okay with that. ___

3. In response to Jill's setting down conditions for your meeting with her parents, you should

    A. Agree with Jill's conditions, saying that you want her to be there. ___

    B. Tell Jill that she can attend if she insists but that you advise against it (i.e., you worry that the anger between her and her mother will undermine the meeting's potential value). ___

    C. Tell her that your purpose is to help her parents understand her better. ___

4. In the aftermath of the family meeting, Jill feels validated but reports that her mother still has made no effort to work on changing herself. You

    A. Give up on conjoint family meetings for the foreseeable future. ___

    B. Give up on any family interventions. ___

    C. Call the mother to encourage her to enter individual therapy. ___

    D. Foster an alliance with the father to support his efforts to buffer the fights between Jill and her mother. ___

    E. Tell her parents that they need to become educated about BPD via books, films, conferences, and organizations. ___

Discussion

1. In response to the parents' inquiry about calling you, you respond

(see "Rationale" and "Family Interventions" in Chapter 7)

A. That you'd like to talk with them but that you will have to get Jill's permission before you will be able to respond to their questions. [3] (This gives Jill too much control. The fact that the parents are financially, legally, and emotionally responsible for Jill gives them rights to be heard. Jill will need to learn to trust your discretion about what should be confidential. The fact that she's been involved in self-endangering behaviors underscores the need for them to be an informed part of Jill's safety net.)

B. That you would like to hear from them if they are concerned about Jill's safety or progress, or about the bills, but cannot discuss what goes on in sessions. [1] (This nicely invites their input but proscribes what you will feel able to discuss.)

C. That you try to keep families involved, so you make yourself available on an as-needed basis. [2] (This sounds good, but it invites them to expect more access than is realistic or than might be in Jill's interest. Jill will need to develop an alliance with you as a trustworthy and wise confidant.)

2. When you learn that Jill's parents didn't follow up on your advice, you should

(see "Basic Therapeutic Approach" in Chapter 2 and "Family Interventions" in Chapter 7)

A. Do nothing. [2] (In the absence of either Jill's or a parental request for more involvement, this is probably the most practical strategy. Still, parental efforts to change often are critical for patients like Jill who are still emotionally and financially dependent on them.)

B. Recognize that her parents are enacting their daughter's primary complaint: they don't want to get involved with her problems. [1] (This is very insightful. Rather than saying this, which might aggravate Jill's anger, it would be more helpful to question Jill's protestations that their lack of follow-up is really okay with her.)

C. Tell Jill that you'd like to follow up on having her parents join a group, but ask whether she's okay with that. [2] (It is good to get Jill's perspective on your doing this. In the absence of complaints, it may make sense to follow Jill's lead, but, still, it will become problematic if these parents don't become educated about Jill's disorder. Their lack of such education adds stress within the home environment and forecloses the possibility of their playing a useful role as collaborators in her treatment.)

3. In response to Jill's setting down conditions for your meeting with her parents, you should

(see "Family Interventions" and "Patient Refuses to Allow Contact With Parents or Spouse" in Chapter 7)

A. Agree with Jill's conditions, saying that you want her to be there. [3] (This would be a good response if her communications with her parents were civil or they all had good control over their anger. There is little reason to expect that those conditions apply here.)

B. Tell Jill that she can attend if she insists but that you advise against it (i.e., you worry that the anger between her and her mother will undermine the meeting's potential value). [1] (This gives her some control, involves her in deciding, but warns her of the potential for unwanted consequences. You can tell Jill that you think her parents will be less defensive toward her after receiving psychoeducation about the disorder's origins, course, and so forth, and recommend that you see them alone.)

C. Tell her that your purpose is to help her parents understand her better. [1] (This is apt to relieve Jill's fears [e.g., that if her parents were to vilify her, you might not be protective]. It helps greatly to clarify your purpose and how it is in your patient's interest. Still, she may not trust you enough yet.)

4. In the aftermath of the family meeting, Jill feels validated but reports that her mother still has made no effort to work on changing herself. You

(see "Family Interventions" in Chapter 7)

A. Give up on conjoint family meetings for the foreseeable future. [1] (Jill and her parents need to change their reactivity to each other before conjoint meetings can be helpful.)

B. Give up on any family interventions. [3] (Conjoint family therapy is premature, but the parents are more likely to be receptive to psychoeducation intervention, and maybe even counseling. They can learn to understand and change their responses to Jill—changes that are more likely to occur without her being present.)

C. Call the mother to encourage her to enter individual therapy. [3] (The mother remains resistant to this idea. Further admonishment might cause her to withdraw from becoming a participant.

She appeared to have opened the door for this therapy [by describing how pained and helpless she feels], and that possibility
might reappear if she becomes less defensive.)

D. Foster an alliance with the father to support his efforts to buffer
the fights between Jill and her mother. [1] (This might be the most
feasible intervention. Dad may be more receptive to the advice
and support from the parents' group than is mother. Inviting him
to come in with Jill and then meeting with the mother separately
are ways to develop an alliance.)

E. Tell her parents that they need to become educated about BPD via
books, films, conferences, and organizations. [1] (Education increases understanding and decreases anger. Some parents can't or
won't change their responses to their BPD child but can be effective advocates on his or her behalf. Provide recommended read-
ings [e.g., "Guidelines for Families"; see Appendix D] or parent
support resources [e.g., Treatment and Research Advancements
Association for Personality Disorder, National Education Alliance
for Borderline Personality Disorder, National Alliance on Mental
Illness].)

SECTION IV

GPM Video Guide
Demonstrations of the Approach

CHAPTER 9
Video Demonstrations

This part of the handbook describes the nine accompanying videos.[1] These videos complement what is prescribed in Section II of this book, "GPM Manual: Treatment Guidelines," and are intended to demonstrate the basic therapeutic approach (see Chapter 2 ["Overall Principles"]) of Good Psychiatric Management (GPM).

Insofar as most of these interactions are scripted to show GPM practices, they necessarily cannot do justice to the need for repetition, the fact that some patients do not respond, and the fact that no clinician, however expert, is always "on model." These excerpts from ongoing therapies can illustrate the intensity and reactivity of the relationships between borderline patients and their treaters, but they can't capture the nuanced quality of each relationship or the remarkable processes in which these relationships have evolved and will continue to change.

1. **Psychoeducation:** This video offers an in vivo example of how basic psychoeducation can be delivered. This interaction is described in the sections "Interpersonal Hypersensitivity" in Chapter 2, "Disclosure of the Diagnosis" in Chapter 3 ("Making the Diagnosis"), "Building an Alliance" in Chapter 6 ("Pharmacotherapy and Comorbidity"), and "Alliance Building" in Chapter 7 ("Split Treatments").

2. **Diagnostic Disclosure:** Here the clinician illustrates a gentle and collaborative way to introduce the borderline personality disorder (BPD) diagnosis. This intervention is described in Chapter 3.

---

[1] The videos can be viewed online by navigating to **www.appi.org/Gunderson** and using the embedded video player. The videos are optimized for most current operating systems, including mobile operating systems iOS 5.1 and Android 4.1 and higher.

3. **Establishing an Alliance:** A clinician works to shift her patient's focus on medications for major depressive disorder (MDD) into a collaborative treatment in which BPD's priority is introduced and the expectations of medications and of the patient's role are changed. The section "Building an Alliance" in Chapter 4 ("Getting Started") and Chapter 6 introduce these issues, elaborated in Case 3, April, in Chapter 8, "Case Illustrations."

4. **Managing Intersession Availability:** This video illustrates a clinician's skillful management of late-night telephone calls, converting an affective crisis into an interpersonal event and introducing the issues of rejection and aloneness. These issues are discussed in the sections "Basic Therapeutic Approach" in Chapter 2 and "Intersession Availability" in Chapter 4. This video has four parts: an office visit, a late-night call, an even later call (both calls are audio only), and the next session. Its issues are illustrated in Case 4, Laura, and Case 5, Lawrence, in Chapter 8.

5. **Managing Safety:** Getting a patient actively involved with protecting his or her own safety is illustrated with GPM's method of creating a safety plan. This video reflects lessons taught in Chapter 2 and in the section "Impending Self-Endangering Behaviors" in Chapter 5 ("Managing Suicidality and Nonsuicidal Self-Harm") and illustrated in Case 2, Loretta, and Case 4, Laura, in Chapter 8.

6. **Managing Anger:** An angry, devaluative patient is calmed only after the clinician interrupts, apologizes for offending, and illustrates both a sense of humor and a persistent focus on the need for the patient to get a job. This video highlights issues from Chapter 2.

7. **Managing Medications:** The clinician illustrates GPM's basic therapeutic principles while trying to both wean the patient from ineffective medications and establish an alliance via pragmatic bargaining. This illustrates the sections "Basic Therapeutic Approach" in Chapter 2 and "General Principles" and "Building an Alliance" in Chapter 6. These issues are also addressed in Case 1, Roger, in Chapter 8.

8. **Managing Safety and Medications:** By requiring an assessment of the baseline frequency of a patient's angry suicidal episodes, the clinician establishes a collaborative alliance vis-à-vis medications. This video illustrates Chapter 6. Case 2, Loretta, and Case 4, Laura, in Chapter 8 illustrate the same issues.

9. **Managing Family Involvement:** This video has four parts. In the first part, a volatile and divisive family has limits set on their anger. The next three segments of the video show each member being seen individually and provided with lessons about BPD and the need to customize their home environment. Chapter 7 describes this. Case 7, Jill, in Chapter 8 dramatizes the same issues.

Appendix A

Relation of Good Psychiatric Management to Other Evidence-Based Treatments for Borderline Personality Disorder

Dialectical Behavior Therapy (DBT)—DBT is a behavior therapy that includes both individual and group therapy and involves didactics and homework on mood monitoring and stress management. It is the best-validated and easiest to learn of the psychotherapies, one that teaches the patient how to regulate feelings and behaviors, with the therapist acting as a coach with extensive availability.

Mentalization-Based Treatment (MBT)—MBT is a cognitive or psychodynamic therapy that uses interventions from self psychology and includes both individual and group therapy. The therapist adopts a "not-knowing" stance while insisting that the patient examine and label his or her own experiences and those of others (i.e., mentalize). Its emphasis on thinking before reacting is probably a process central to all effective therapies.

Transference-Focused Psychotherapy (TFP)—TFP is a twice-weekly individual psychotherapy developed within the object relations psychoanalytic theory. It includes interpretation of motives or feelings unknown to the patient and retains a focus on the patient's misunderstanding of others, especially of the therapist (i.e., transference). It is the least supportive and hardest to learn of the therapies.

Adapted from Gunderson JG: "Clinical Practice: Borderline Personality Disorder." *New England Journal of Medicine* 26:2037–2042, 2011.

Comparative Features

Therapy	Model	Intensity (hours/week)	Duration	Modalities	Focus	Validation[a]	Managing S/SI
DBT	Emotional dysregulation	~3	1 year	Individual and group	Feelings and SIB	+++	Skills, 24/7 cvg
MBT	Misunderstood mental states	~3	1.5 year	Individual and group	Cognitions and feelings	++	Emergency department
TFP	Unintegrated aggression	~2	1 year	Individual	Interpersonal	+	Emergency department
GPM	Interpersonal hypersensitivity	~1–2	As needed	Individual/ medications and group, family	Interpersonal and social	+	Contingent, not 24/7 cvg

Note. S/SI = suicidality/suicidal ideation; SIB = self-injurious behavior; cvg = coverage (on call).
DBT = Dialectical Behavior Therapy; MBT = Mentalization-Based Treatment; TFP = Transference-Focused Psychotherapy; GPM = Good Psychiatric Management.
[a]Validation = level of empirical support (+++ = very strong, ++ = strong, + = modest).

Good Psychiatric Management's Specificity

- Case management versus psychotherapy
- Focus on situations, interpersonal stressors, and vocation (i.e., work is prioritized over love)
- Emphasis on psychoeducation integrating genetics, course, and quest for caregiving
- View of the therapy relationship itself as corrective
- Integration of medication, family involvement, and other modalities

GPM is a treatment that rests firmly on the shoulders of others. The first major influence was Otto Kernberg's major clinical and theoretical contributions and their gradual elaboration in TFP. This model encouraged a focus on the borderline patient's aggression and the failures to integrate it. From this perspective, I (the first author) learned to monitor countertransference, guard boundaries, hold patients accountable for their avoidance and acting out, and, perhaps most specifically, realize the value of interpretation. I still hold these lessons dear, but in practice I found that TFP was often insufficiently supportive. The self psychology paradigm applied to BPD by Adler (1986) proved more palatable to patients. It emphasized the importance of alliance building, the value of validation, and the significance of corrective experience within the therapeutic relationship. The introduction of behavior modification theory and its application to BPD as DBT by Linehan (1993) openly challenged the prevailing psychoanalytic models. Although behavior modification was foreign to my training, I quickly observed that DBT openly endorsed practices I know were necessary and useful—practices such as coaching, reassurances, and contingencies that were not found within psychoanalytic models. It also introduced the idea that the misadventures of borderline patients could derive from a lack of social skills—not from conflict. Interventions such as didactics, skills training, and homework were great additions.

Anthony Bateman and Peter Fonagy's MBT (1999) model of treatment for BPD explicitly was thought to correct empirically observed early developmental failures in caregiving. This was conceptually and clinically innovative. MBT, like DBT, saw borderline patients as lacking skills, but unlike in DBT, the skill deficits were in reading their own and others' minds. MBT emphasized the clinician's role as a curious "not-knowing" explorer. This model underscores the importance of self-awareness and empathy and therapy's core role in correcting misattributions.

Appendix B

Common Features of Evidence-Based Treatments for Borderline Personality Disorder

Primary clinician—Designation of one clinician to discuss the diagnosis with the patient, assess progress, monitor safety, and oversee communications with other practitioners and family members.

Structure—Establishment of goals and roles, limits of clinician availability, and a plan for managing suicidal or other emergencies.

Support—Concerned attention; validation of the patient's distress, desperation, and hopeful potential for change.

Involvement—Progress depends on the patient's active efforts to take control over his or her feelings and behavior.

Active interventions—Clinicians need to be active (interrupt silences and digressions); focus on here-and-now situations (including angry or dismissive responses); and help the patient connect his or her feelings to rejections, lost supports, and other events.

Concerned nonreactive responses to suicidal threats or self-harm—Clinicians convey concern but react judiciously (i.e., not always recommending hospitalization) and discuss with colleagues.

Self-awareness—Idealization or devaluation inclines clinicians to rescue or punish, respectively (countertransference); such responses require discussion with colleagues.

Adapted from Bateman 2012; Gunderson 2011; and Weinberg et al. 2011.

Appendix C

Safety Planning: An Example

The patient whose safety plan (see pp. 39 and 42) is shown on the next page is a 53-year-old divorced mother of one with a diagnosis of borderline personality disorder and a history of major depression and current social phobia. She came to the attention of psychiatry at a somewhat older age, having relatively minor self-harm behaviors and, in more recent years, some low-lethality overdose attempts. The patient had been seen several times in emergency departments after overdosing on small amounts of medication. Her self-harm behaviors are often precipitated by arguments with her adult daughter. Development of the patient's safety plan is shown in Video 5: Managing Safety, described in Chapter 9, "Video Demonstrations."

Adapted from Stanley B, Brown GK: "Safety Planning Interventions: A Brief Intervention to Mitigate Suicide Risk." *Cognitive and Behavioral Practice* 19:256–264, 2012.

Safety Plan

Step 1: Warning Signs.

* Feeling panicky
* Feeling I can't breathe; wanting to get out
* Wanting to take pills or drink

Step 2: Coping Using Distraction or Soothing Strategies.

* Petting my dog

Step 3: Social Situations or People Who Can Help Distract Me.

* Two girlfriends can be helpful.

Step 4: People I Can Ask for Help.
(Note if a person is unhelpful when you are in crisis.)

* Do not ask my mother for help during a crisis.

Step 5: Professionals or Agencies I Can Contact During a Crisis.

* "COAST" crisis phone line
* List of others to be completed as homework

Step 6: Making the Environment Safer.

* Lock my medications up so that they are not readily available.

Appendix D
Guidelines for Families

Goals: Go Slowly

1. Remember that change is difficult to achieve and the prospect of it is fraught with fears. Be cautious about suggesting that "great" progress has been made or giving "you can do it" reassurances. "Progress" evokes fears of abandonment.
2. Lower your expectations. Set realistic goals that are available. Solve big problems in small steps. Work on one thing at a time. "Big" goals or long-term goals lead to discouragement and failure.

Family Environment: Keep Things Cool

1. Keep things cool and calm. Appreciation is normal. Tone it down. Disagreement is normal. Tone it down, too.
2. Maintain family routines as much as possible. Stay in touch with family and friends. There's more to life than problems, so don't give up the good times.
3. Find time to talk. Chats about light or neutral matters are helpful. Schedule times for this if you need to.

Adapted from Gunderson J, Berkowitz C: *Family Guidelines: Multiple Family Group Program at McLean Hospital.* New England Personality Disorder Association. Available at: http://www.borderlinepersonalitydisorder.com/wp-content/uploads/2012/10/Palmer_NEABPD10_14_12a-1.pdf. Accessed May 2, 2013.

Managing Crises:
Pay Attention But Stay Calm

1. Don't get defensive in the face of accusations and criticisms. However unfair these may be, say little and don't fight. Allow yourself to be hurt. Admit to whatever is true in the criticisms.
2. Self-destructive acts or threats require attention. Don't ignore them. Don't panic. Don't keep secrets about this. Talk about it openly with your family member and make sure professionals know.
3. Listen. People need to have their negative feelings heard. Don't say "it isn't so." Don't try to make the feelings go away. Using words to express fear, loneliness, inadequacy, anger, or needs is good. It is better to use words than to act on feelings.

Addressing Problems:
Collaborate and Be Consistent

1. When solving a family member's problems, ALWAYS
   a. Involve the family member in identifying what needs to be done.
   b. Ask whether the person can "do" what is needed in the solution.
   c. Ask whether the person wants you to help him or her "do" what is needed.
2. Family members need to act in concert with one another. Parental inconsistencies fuel severe family conflicts. Develop strategies that everyone can stick to.
3. If you have concerns about medications or therapist interventions, make sure that both your family member and his or her therapist or doctor know. If you have financial responsibility, you have the right to address your concerns to the therapist or doctor.

Limit Setting: Be Direct But Careful

1. Set limits by stating the limits of your tolerance. Let your expectations be known in clear, simple language. Everyone needs to know what is expected of them.
2. Do not protect family members from the natural consequences of their actions. Allow them to learn about reality. Bumping into a few walls is usually necessary.

3. Do not tolerate abusive treatment such as tantrums, threats, hitting, and spitting. Walk away and return to discuss the issue later.

4. Be cautious about using threats and ultimatums. They are a last resort. Do not use threats and ultimatums as a means of convincing others to change. Present them only when you can and will carry through. Let others—including professionals—help you decide when to give them.

References

Adler G: Borderline Psychopathology and Its Treatment. New York, Jason Aronson, 1986

American Psychiatric Association Practice Guidelines: Practice guideline for the treatment of patients with borderline personality disorder. American Psychiatric Association. Am J Psychiatry 158:1–52, 2001

Bateman A: Treating borderline personality disorder in clinical practice. Am J Psychiatry 169:560–563, 2012

Bateman A, Fonagy P: The effectiveness of partial hospitalization in the treatment of BPD: a randomized controlled trial. Am J Psychiatry 156:1563–1569, 1999

Bateman A, Fonagy P: Randomized controlled trial of outpatient mentalization-based treatment versus structured clinical management for borderline personality disorder. Am J Psychiatry 166:1355–1364, 2009

Bateman AW, Fonagy P: Handbook of Mentalizing in Mental Health Practice. Washington, DC, American Psychiatric Publishing, 2012

Bender DS, Skodol AE, Pagano ME, et al: Prospective assessment of treatment use by patients with personality disorders. Psychiatr Serv 57: 254–257, 2006

Chanen AM, Jackson HJ, McCutcheon LK, et al: Early intervention for adolescents with borderline personality disorder using cognitive analytic therapy: randomized controlled trial. Br J Psychiatry 193:477–484, 2008

Clarkin JF, Levy KN, Lenzenweger MF, et al: Evaluating three treatments for borderline personality disorder: a multiwave study. Am J Psychiatry 164:922–928, 2007

Cloud J: The mystery of borderline personality disorder. Time Magazine. January 19, 2009, Vol 173, No 2.

Cowdry RW, Gardner DL: Pharmacotherapy of borderline personality disorder: alprazolam, carbamazepine, trifluoperazine, and tranylcypromine. Arch Gen Psychiatry 45:111–119, 1988

Dawson D, MacMillan HL: Relationship Management and the Borderline Patient. New York, Brunner/Mazel, 1993

Donegan NH, Sanislow CA, Blumberg HP, et al: Amygdala hyperreactivity in borderline personality disorder: implications for emotional dysregulation. Biol Psychiatry 54:1285–1293, 2003

Gabbard GO: Do all roads lead to Rome? New findings on borderline personality disorder. Am J Psychiatry 164:922–928, 2007

Grilo CM, Sanislow CA, Skodol AE, et al: Longitudinal diagnostic efficiency of DSM-IV criteria for borderline personality disorder: a two-year prospective study. Can J Psychiatry 52:357–362, 2007

Gunderson JG: Borderline Personality Disorder: A Clinical Guide. Washington, DC, American Psychiatric Press, 1984

Gunderson JG: The borderline patient's intolerance of aloneness: insecure attachments and therapist availability. Am J Psychiatry 153:752–758, 1996

Gunderson JG: Borderline Personality Disorder: A Clinical Guide. Washington, DC, American Psychiatric Press, 2001

Gunderson JG: Disturbed relationships as a phenotype for borderline personality disorder. Am J Psychiatry 164:1637–1640, 2007

Gunderson JG: Borderline personality disorder: ontogeny of a diagnosis. Am J Psychiatry 166:530–539, 2009

Gunderson JG: Clinical practice: borderline personality disorder. N Engl J Med 26:2037–2042, 2011

Gunderson JG, Berkowitz CB: Family Guidelines: Multiple Family Group Program at McLean Hospital. Belmont, MA, New England Personality Disorder Association, 2006. http://www.borderlinepersonalitydisorder.com/wp-content/uploads/2012/10/Palmer_NEABPD10_14_12a-1.pdf. Accessed May 2, 2013.

Gunderson JG, Links P: Borderline Personality Disorder: A Clinical Guide, 2nd Edition. Washington, DC, American Psychiatric Publishing, 2008

Gunderson JG, Lyons-Ruth K: BPD's interpersonal hypersensitivity phenotype: a gene-environment-developmental model. J Pers Disord 22:22–41, 2008

Gunderson JG, Bender D, Sanislow C, et al: Plausibility and possible determinants of sudden "remissions" in borderline patients. Psychiatry 66:111–119, 2003

Gunderson JG, Morey LC, Stout RL, et al: Major depressive disorder and borderline personality disorder revisited: longitudinal interactions. J Clin Psychiatry 65:1049–1056, 2004

Gunderson JG, Stout RL, McGlashan TH, et al: Ten-year course of borderline personality disorder: psychopathology and function: from the Collaborative Longitudinal Personality Disorders study. Arch Gen Psychiatry 68:827–837, 2011

Gunderson JG, Stout RI, Keuroghlian A, Shea MT, Keuroghlian A, Morey LC, Grilo CM, Sanislow C, Yen S, Zanarini MC, Markowitz JC, McGlashan TH, Skodol AE: Interactions of borderline personality disorder with affective disorders. Paper presented at the 165th annual meeting of the American Psychiatric Association, Philadelphia, PA, May 5–9, 2012

Keuroghlian A: Interactions of borderline personality disorder and anxiety disorders, eating disorders, and substance use disorders over 10 years. Paper presented at American Psychiatric Association 166th annual meeting, San Francisco, CA, May 18, 2013

Kolla NJ, Links PS, McMain S: Demonstrating adherence to guidelines for the treatment of patients with borderline personality disorder. Can J Psychiatry 54(3):181–189, 2009

Linehan MM: Dialectical Behavioral Therapy of Borderline Personality Disorder. New York, Guilford, 1993

Links PS, Kolla N: Assessing and managing suicide risk, in The American Psychiatric Publishing Textbook of Personality Disorders. Edited by Oldham JM, Skodol AE, Bender DS. Washington, DC, American Psychiatric Publishing, 2005, pp 449–462

Maltsberger JT, Ronningstam E, Weinberg I, et al: Suicide fantasy as a life-sustaining recourse. J Am Acad Psychoanal Dyn Psychiatry 38:611–623, 2011

McGlashan TH: Implications of outcome research for the treatment of borderline personality disorder, in Borderline Personality Disorder: Etiology and Treatment. Edited by Paris J. Washington, DC, American Psychiatric Press, 1993, pp 235–260

McMain SF, Links PS, Gnam WH, et al: A randomized trial of dialectical behavior therapy versus general psychiatric management for borderline personality disorder. Am J Psychiatry 166:1–10, 2009

McMain SF, Guimond T, Streiner DL, et al: Dialectical behavior therapy compared with general psychiatric management for borderline personality disorder: clinical outcomes and functioning over a 2-year follow-up. Am J Psychiatry 169: 650–661, 2012

Mercer D, Douglass AB, Links PS: Meta-analyses of mood stabilizers, antidepressants and antipsychotics in the treatment of borderline personality disorder: effectiveness for depression and anger symptoms. J Pers Disord 23:156–174, 2009

Nadort M, Arntz A, Smit JH, et al: Implementation of outpatient schema therapy for borderline personality disorder with versus without crisis support by the therapist outside office hours: a randomized trial. Behav Res Ther 47:961–973, 2009

Rockland LH: A supportive approach: psychodynamically oriented supportive therapy: treatment of borderline patients who self-mutilate. J Pers Disord 1:350–353, 1987

Rockland LH: Supportive Therapy for Borderline Patients: A Psychodynamic Approach. New York, Guilford, 1992

Shanks C, Pfohl B, Blum N, et al: Can negative attitudes toward patients with borderline personality disorder be changed? The effect of attending a STEPPES workshop. J Pers Disord 25:806–812, 2011

Silbersweig D, Clarkin JF, Goldstein M, et al: Failure of frontolimbic inhibitory function in the context of negative emotion in borderline personality disorder. Am J Psychiatry 164:1832–1841, 2007

Silk KR, Faurino L: Psychopharmacology of personality disorders, in The Oxford Handbook of Personality Disorders. Edited by Widiger T. London, England, Oxford University Press, 2012, pp 712–726

Stanley B, Gameroff MJ, Michalsen V, et al: Are suicide attempters who self-mutilate a unique population? Am J Psychiatry 158:427–432, 2001

Weinberg I, Ronningstam E, Goldblatt MJ, et al: Common factors in empirically supported treatments of borderline personality disorder. Curr Psychiatry Rep 13:60–68, 2011

Winnicott DW: Transitional objects and transitional phenomena: a study of the first not-me possession. Int J Psychoanal 34:89–97, 1953

Yen S, Shea MT, Sanislow CA, et al: Borderline personality disorder criteria associated with prospectively observed suicidal behavior. Am J Psychiatry 161:1296–1298, 2004

Yen S, Pagano ME, Shea MT, et al: Recent life events preceding suicide attempts in a personality disorder sample: findings from the collaborative longitudinal personality disorders study. J Consult Clin Psychol 73:99–105, 2005

Yen S, Shea MT, Sanislow CA, et al: Personality traits as prospective predictors of suicide attempts. Acta Psychiatr Scand 120:222–229, 2009

Yeomans FE, Clarkin JF, Kernberg OF: A Primer for Transference Focused Psychotherapy for the Borderline Patient. Northvale, NJ, Jason Aronson, 2002

Young JE: Cognitive Therapy for Personality Disorders. Sarasota, FL, Professional Resource Exchange, 1990

Zanarini MC, Frankenburg FR, DeLuca CJ, et al: The pain of being borderline: dysphoric states specific to borderline personality disorder. Harv Rev Psychiatry 6:201–207, 1998

Zanarini MC, Frankenburg FR, Reich DB, et al: Time to attainment of recovery from borderline personality disorder and stability of recovery: a 10-year prospective follow-up study. Am J Psychiatry 167:663–667, 2010

Index

Page numbers printed in *boldface* type refer to tables or figures.

AA. *See* Alcoholics Anonymous
Active interventions, as common
 feature of evidence-based
 treatments for BPD, 149
Adler, Gerald, 147
Alcoholics Anonymous (AA), 58
Anger, management of, video
 demonstration, 144
Anorexia, comorbidity with BPD, **53**
Antipsychotics
 symptom targets, **51**
 for treatment of BPD, 50, **50**
Antisocial personality disorder,
 comorbidity with BPD, **53**
Anxiolytics
 symptom targets, **51**
 for treatment of BPD, 52
Availability, of clinician to patient
 intersession, 28–30, **31**
 managing unavailability, 35
 safety of patient and, 84

Bateman, Anthony, 147
Bipolar disorder, comorbidity with
 BPD, **53,** 55
Borderline personality disorder (BPD)
 algorithm for medication choice,
  50
 attitudes toward treating a patient
  with, vii
 building an alliance, 30–33
  sequential forms of therapeutic
   alliance, **32**
  video demonstration, 144

case examples
 of anxiety and depression, 78–86
 of comorbidities, 72–78
 of failed split treatment, 128–
  134
 of family interventions, 134–139
 of hospitalization and
  dependency, 95–104
 of long-term management, 104–
  128
 making the diagnosis, 72–78
 of somatization and alliance
  building, 87–95
change in patient, 18–20
changing therapists, 33–34
common features of evidence-based
 treatments for, 149
comorbidities, 52, **53**
 case example of, 72–78
current status of pharmacotherapy
 for, **49**
diagnosis of, 21–25
 as basis for developing a
  treatment alliance, 22
 case example of, 72–78
 disclosure, 21–23
 how to disclose, 23–24
 preparation for clinician, 22
disclosure, 23–24
flexibility of clinician, 18
Good Psychiatric Management for,
 3–10
guidelines for families of a patient
 with, 153–155

Borderline personality disorder (BPD)
(*continued*)
interpersonal coherence, 13, **14**
life outside of treatment, 17–18
myths about treatment of, **viii**
patient accountability, 17
patient refusal of diagnosis of, 24
pharmacotherapy, 47–55
building an alliance, 48–49
comorbidities, 52, **53**
general principles of, 47–48
problems with, 54–55
bipolar disorder and, 55
depression and, 55
mood stabilizers and, 55
patient refusal of
medications, 54
patient resistance to
discontinuing
medications, 54
use of medications for
agitated or self-harming
patient, 54
selection of medications, 49–52
psychoeducation for patient and
patient's family, **23**
randomized controlled trials of
specific therapies for, 6
relation of GPM to other evidence-
based treatments for, 145–147
relationships with patient with, viii
safety planning for the patient with,
151–152
video demonstration, 144
self-disclosure by clinicians in
treatment of, **17**
social rehabilitation of patient with,
19, **19**
split treatments, 57–67
common problems, 58–60
communication with
physician, 59
co-treater and, 60
patient devalues the other
treater, 58–59

complementary functions of
different modalities, **59**
family interventions, 62–67
alliance building, 63–65
collaboration, 65
common problems, 65–67
hierarchy, **64**
parental participation, 63
patient support for parent
or spouse participation,
63
psychoeducation, 64–65
framework for, **58**
group therapy, 60–61
absences from, 62
case example of, 104–128
exclusionary alliances
between group
members, 62
hierarchy of, **61**
nonparticipatory behaviors
within sessions, 62
rationale, 57
selection of another modality,
57–58, **59**
suicide as symptom of, 37–45
treatment, establishment of, 27–35
case example of, 72–78
clinician unavailability to
patient, 35
intersession availability, 28–30
medications, 32
patient cannot relate to treater,
34–35
patient refusal to accept
framework, 34
progress, assessment of, 28
treatment centers, specialized, 4–5
BPD. *See* Borderline Personality
Disorder
Bulimia, comorbidity with BPD, **53**

Case examples
of anxiety and depression, 78–86
case vignette, 78–80

decision points/alternative
responses, 80–82
discussion, 82–86
of comorbidities, 72–78
case vignette, 72–73
decision points/alternative
responses, 73–74
discussion, 75–78
of establishing an alliance, 87–95
case vignette, 87–89
decision points/alternative
responses, 89–90
discussion, 91–95
overview, 87
of failed split treatment, 128–134
case vignette, 128–129
decision points/alternative
responses, 129–130
discussion, 131–134
overview, 128
of family interventions, 134–139
case vignette, 134–135
decision points/alternative
responses, 135–136
discussion, 137–139
overview, 134
of hospitalization and dependency,
95–104
case vignette, 96–97
decision points/alternative
responses, 97–99
discussion, 99–104
overview, 95
of long-term therapy, 104–128
case vignettes, 104–111
decision points/alternative
responses, 111–116
discussion, 116–128
overview, 104
making the diagnosis, 72–78
overview, 71
of selection of appropriate level of
care, 104–128
of somatization and alliance
building, 87–95

case vignette, 87–89
decision points/alternative
responses, 89–90
discussion, 91–95
Case management, **59**
with GPM, **7**
CAT. *See* Cognitive Analytic Therapy
Chain analysis, 33
Chlorpromazine, 54
Clinicians
alliance building with patient,
87–95
changing therapists, 33–34
clinician-patient relationship, 16,
30–31, 35
video demonstration, 144
colleagues of, 41
communication with, 59
corrective experiences of, 20
diagnosis of borderline personality
disorder for preparation of
treatment, 22
disclosure versus nondisclosure of
diagnosis of borderline
personality disorder, **22**
encouragement of patient, 18–19
flexibility of, 18
limits of, 41
managing intersession availability,
video demonstration, 144
message of "work before love,"
17–18
patient refusal to allow clinician to
contact significant others,
44–45
role in completed suicide,
42–43
self-disclosure by clinicians in
treatment, **17**
unavailability to patient, 35
Cognitive Analytic Therapy (CAT),
and GPM, 6
Common features, of evidence-based
treatments for BPD, 149
Counseling, **64**

DBT. *See* Dialectical Behavior Therapy

Depression, BPD and, 55

Diagnostic disclosure, video
    demonstration, 143

Dialectical Behavior Therapy (DBT), 61
  comparative features of, **146**
  description of, 145
  GPM and, 4–5
  integration with GPM, **8**

Dichotomous stance, 48

DSM, threshold for diagnosis of BPD,
    24–25

Eating disorder, comorbidity with BPD,
    53

Eating Disorders Anonymous, 58

Establishing an alliance, video
    demonstration, 144

Family interventions, **59,** 62–67, 134–
    139
  alleged sexual or physical abuse
    within family, 66
  alliance building, 63–65
    collaboration, 65
    psychoeducation, 64–65
    support, 63–64
  estranged parents, 67
  fear of suicide or self-harm, 66
  guidelines for, 153–155
    collaboration and consistency, 154
    family environment, 153.
    goals, 153
    limit setting, 154–155
    managing crises, 154
  hierarchy, **64**
  intake session with the patient, 63
  parental disinterest or disrespect,
    66–67
  parental participation, 63
  patient refusal to allow contact with
    parents or spouse, 65–66
  patient support for parent or spouse
    participation, 63
  video demonstration, 144

Family therapy, **64**

Fonagy, Peter, 147

General Psychiatric Management, as
    research "brand," 8–10. *See also*
    Good Psychiatric Management
    (GPM), empirical validation of

Goals, setting, 33

"Good enough," concept, ix
  clinician availability for patient's
    safety and, 84
  clinician competence to treat BPD
    and, vii–viii, ix, 3–4, 52
  GPM and, 4–5
  patient's sense of self and, 13

Good Psychiatric Management (GPM),
    ix, 3–10. *See also* General
    Psychiatric Management
  active versus reactive, 15
  basic therapeutic approach, 15–18
  building an alliance, 30–33
  change in patient, 16–17
  changing therapists, 33–34
  characteristics, distinct, 7
  comparative features of, 5, **8, 146**
  empirical validation of, 8–10
  integration of prior evidence-based
    psychotherapies, **8**
  interpersonal hypersensitivity
    theory and, **7,** 13–20
  intersession availability, 28–30, **31**
  overview, 3–4
  patient-clinician relations, 16, 30–
    31, 35
  precedents and foundations of, 5–7
  principles of, 13–20, **16**
  progress assessment of, 28
  psychoeducation, **7,** 15
  relation to other evidence-based
    treatments for BPD, 4–5, **8,**
    145–147
  research-based endorsement of, 10
  self-disclosure by clinicians in
    treatment, **17**
  setting the framework, 27–28, **28**

overview, 27
patient cannot relate to, 34–35
patient refusal to accept, 34
specificity of, 147
therapeutic alliance, sequential
    forms of **32**
therapeutic processes, **19**
therapy relationship, 16
thoughtfulness, 15
as treatment model, 6–7
treatment planning and, 4–5
    progress assessment of, 28, **30**
    setting goals, 33
GPM. *See* Good Psychiatric
    Management
Group therapy, **59**
absences from, 62
case example of, 104–128
exclusionary alliances between
    group members, 62
hierarchy of, **61**
nonparticipatory behaviors within
    sessions, 62
skills training groups, 61

Homework, as alliance builder,
    32–33

Interpersonal hypersensitivity
and GPM, **7**, 13–20
and "holding environment," 13
Interventions
active, 149
family, 62–67
    case example, 134–139
psychoeducation for, 64–65, **64**
Involvement, as common feature of
    evidence-based treatments for
    BPD, 149

Kernberg, Otto, 147

Language, examples of, for use in
    psychoeducation
for disclosing the diagnosis, 23–24

for educating patient about
    "disconnection," 34
for endorsing group therapy, 60
for managing family involvement,
    62–63, 64–65
for managing intersession
    availability, 28
for managing safety of a suicidal
    patient, 38, 44
for managing medications, 48
for setting the framework, 27
Liability concerns, and importance
    of involving colleagues, 37, **39**,
    41
Linehan, Marsha, 147
Links, Paul S., 9

Major depressive disorder, comorbidity
    with BPD, **53**, 55
MBT. *See* Mentalization-Based
    Treatment
McGlashan, Thomas H., 6
McLean Hospital, as example of
    tertiary care treatment center for
    BPD, 5
McMain, Shelley, 8, 9
Medications. *See also*
    Pharmacotherapy
selection of, 49–52
Mentalization-Based Treatment
    (MBT)
comparative features of, **146**
description of, 145
GPM and, 5
integration with good psychiatric
    management, **8**
Model, of Good Psychiatric
    Management for treatment, 6–7
Mood stabilizers
symptom targets, **51**
for treatment of BPD, 49, 55

Narcissistic personality disorder,
    comorbidity with BPD, **53**
Narcotics Anonymous, 58

Olanzapine, 54

Panic disorder, comorbidity with BPD,
    53
Parents
    disinterest in or disrespect of
        patient, 66–67
    estranged, 67
    participation in family intervention,
        63
    patient refusal to allow contact
        with, 65–66
Patient
    accountability of, 17
    cannot relate to treatment, 34–35
    changes in, 16–17, 18–20
    clinician-patient relationship, 16,
        30–31, 35
        video demonstration, 144
    collaboration with
        pharmacotherapy, 48
    corrective experiences of, **19**
    disclosure versus nondisclosure of
        diagnosis of BPD, **22**
    DSM threshold for diagnosis, 24–
        25
    expectations about diagnosis of
        course of BPD, 21, **22**
    homework for, 32–33
    hospitalization for suicidality, 44
    intake session with, 63
    life outside of treatment, 17–18
    negative attitudes toward
        pharmacotherapy, 48–49
    progress assessment of, 28
    recurrence of suicide attempts, 43
    refusal of diagnosis of BPD, 24
    refusal of medications, 54
    refusal to accept treatment, 34
    refusal to allow clinician to contact
        significant others, 44–45
    refusal to take suicide "off the
        table," 45
    resistance to discontinuing
        medications, 54

selection of appropriate level of
        care, 39–40, **41**
    social rehabilitation of, 19, **19**
    thinking before acting, 18–19, **19**
    treatment establishment, 27–35
        intersession availability, 30–31, **31**
        progress assessment of, **30**
    use of medications for agitated or
        self-harming patient, 54
Pharmacotherapy, 47–55. *See also*
    Medications
    algorithm for medication choice for
        BPD, **50**
    avoidance of dichotomous stance,
        48
    case examples of, 72–78, 78–86,
        87–95
    communication with clinician, 59
    comorbidity and, 72–78
    current status for BPD, **49**
    managing medications, video
        demonstration, 144
    patient collaboration with, 48
    selection of medications, 49–52
Physical abuse, 66
Posttraumatic stress disorder,
    comorbidity with BPD, **53**
Primary clinician, designation of, as
    common feature of evidence-
    based treatments for BPD, 149
Psychoeducation. *See also* Language,
    examples of, for use in
    psychoeducation
    for building an alliance, 48
    for family interventions, 64–65, **64**
    in GPM, **7,** 15
    for parameters for hopefulness and
        patient participation, 31
    for patient and patient's family, **23**
    video demonstration, 143
Psychotherapy, **59**
    integration of prior evidence-
        based, **8**

Quetiapine, 54

Safety
    planning, 39, 42, 151
    video demonstration, 144
Selective serotonin reuptake inhibitors
        (SSRIs)
    symptom targets, **51**
    for treatment of BPD, 49
Self-awareness, by clinician, as
        common feature of evidence-
        based treatments for BPD, 149
Self-harm
    aftermath of self-endangering
        behaviors, 42–43
    case examples of, 78–86, 104–
        128
    concerned nonreactive responses
        to, 149
    family fear of, 66
    liability concerns in treatment of
        patient, **39**
    overview, 37
    patient refusal to allow clinician to
        contact significant others,
        44–45
    patient refusal to decrease self-harm
        behaviors, 45
    selection of appropriate level of
        care, 39–40, **40, 41**
    self-endangering behaviors and,
        38–41
        assessment of, 38–39
    as symptom of BPD, 37–45, **38**
Self-help organizations, **58, 59**
Sexual abuse, 66
Skills training groups, 61
Social rehabilitation, 19, **19**
Somatization, case example of, 87–
    95
Spouse, patient refusal to allow contact
        with, 65–66
SSRIs. *See* Selective serotonin reuptake
        inhibitors
Structure, establishment of, as
        common feature of evidence-
        based treatments for BPD, 149

Substance use disorder, comorbidity
        with BPD, **53**
Suicide, 37–45
    acute-on-chronic risk of, **40**
    aftermath of self-endangering
        behaviors, 42–43
    case example of suicidality, 78–86
    completed, 42–43
    concerned nonreactive responses to
        suicidal threats or self-harm,
        as common feature of
        evidence-based treatments for
        BPD, 149
    family fear of, 66
    hospitalization of patient, 44
    overview, 37
    patient refusal to take suicide "off
        the table," 45
    recurrence of attempts, 37, 43
    selection of appropriate level of
        care, 39–40, 41, **40**
    self-endangering behaviors and,
        38–41
        assessment of, **38–39**
    as symptom of BPD, **37–45, 38**
    unsuccessful attempts, 42–43
        future safety issues, 42
Support, as common feature of
        evidence-based treatments for
        BPD, 149
Support groups, **64**

TCAs. *See* Tricyclic antidepressants
TFP. *See* Transference-Focused
        Psychotherapy
Therapy, clinician-patient relationship,
        16, 30–31, 35
Transference-Focused Psychotherapy
        (TFP)
    comparative features of, **146**
    description of, 145
    GPM and, 5
    integration with GPM, **8**
Tricyclic antidepressants (TCAs), for
        treatment of BPD, 49

Videos
  of diagnostic disclosure, 143
  of establishing an alliance, 144
  of managing anger, 144
  of managing family involvement,
    144
  of managing intersession
    availability, 144
  of managing medications, 144
  of managing safety, 144
  of managing safety and medications,
    144
  of psychoeducation, 143

Winnicott, D.W., ix